100 SMART CHOICES

EASY IDEAS FOR LIVING HEALTHIER AND HAPPIER

Michael W. Rosen, MD, Medical Consultant

This book was published by OptumHealth℠ in partnership with Rodale Inc., publisher of *Prevention, Men's Health* and *Women's Health*.

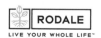

RODALE
LIVE YOUR WHOLE LIFE™

100 Smart Choices is intended as a reference guide only, not as a medical manual. The information given here is designed to help you make informed decisions about your health. It is not intended as a substitute for any treatment that may have been prescribed by your doctor. If you suspect that you have a medical problem, we urge you to seek competent medical help.

Mention of specific companies, organizations or authorities in this book does not imply endorsement by the author or publisher, nor does mention of specific companies, organizations or authorities imply that they endorse this book, its author or the publisher.

Internet addresses and telephone numbers given in this book were accurate at the time it went to press.

Printed in the United States of America on acid-free, recycled paper.

Library of Congress Cataloging-in-Publication Data

Rosen, Michael W.
100 smart choices / Michael W. Rosen
p. cm.
ISBN-13 978-1-60529-750-7 paperback
ISBN-10 1-60529-750-X paperback
1. Health—Popular works. 2. Self-care, Health—Popular works. 3. Medicine, Preventive—Popular works. I. Title. II. Title: One hundred smart choices.
RA776.R733 2008
613—dc22   2008040858

OptumHealth℠

Lead Medical Consultants

Medical Director
Michael W. Rosen, MD

Medical Consultant
Phyllis DeCarlo Cross, MD, MPH

Medical Consultant
Tanise I. Edwards, MD, FAAEM

Contributing Medical Consultants

Senior Manager, Clinical Services
Nancy Berryman, RN

Director, Medical-Behavioral Integration
Arleen Fitzgerald, MSW, LICSW

Consulting Nutritionist
Melanie Polk, MMSc, RD, FADA

Dental Consultant
Lee R. Shapiro, DMD

Vice President Clinical Product Development
Michael Weitzner, DMD, MS

Editorial Consultants

Creative Director, the Carrot agency
Sara Fitzgerald Sonntag

Associate Creative Director, the Carrot agency
Kate Ranta Maffei

Business Managers

Vice President Product Management, Wellness
Sean P. McNattin

Director Product Management, Wellness
Jason P. Lee, MBA

Publications Product Manager
Amber Gunn Thomas

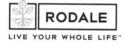 **Prevention**

Rodale Custom Publishing

Executive Editors
Debra Witt, Jennifer Leight

Editor
Cheryl Winters-Tetreau

Fact Checkers
Traci Stocker
Adrien Drozdowski

Copy Editors
Robert Williams
Kathleen Paton

Designers
Stephanie Thompson
Amanda Benfer
T.J. Harkins

Senior Vice President/Publisher
Valerie Valente

Director of Publishing
Duncan Milne

Vice President/Editorial Director
Nelson Peña

Creative Director
Carol Pagliuco

Account Director
Janice Miller

Associate Publisher Marketing
Marcie Avram

Production/Services Specialist
Jodi Schaffer

CONTENTS

100 SMART CHOICES

Wellness Boosters

Smart Choices Today for a Healthier Tomorrow

Symptom Solutions

How to Make Smart Health Care Choices

CONTENTS

100 SMART CHOICES

15 SMART CHOICES Take-Charge Tools

Get Equipped to Make Smart Choices

TO OUR READERS

AS THE TITLE SUGGESTS, THIS BOOK GETS TO THE heart of smart health choices that can give you the greatest return—peace of mind. Peace of mind that you are taking the right steps toward better health. Comfort in knowing how to get the best care when you need it most. Confidence that you are taking charge of your health and medical care.

Part One focuses on lifestyle changes where even small changes can make a big difference in your overall health. We hope that you will follow the advice regarding eating well, staying active, relieving stress and more.

Part Two provides helpful suggestions that can guide you as you make smart decisions about your medical care. For example, you will find useful information on how to distinguish between true emergencies and less serious symptoms.

When a health issue arises, this section will help you understand your symptoms and make more informed intervention decisions.

Part Three provides a variety of convenient tools that will help you put all of these smart choices into *action!* Track your progress toward your wellness goals. Record past medical care. And, plan preventive care for the future.

We are excited to provide you with *100 Smart Choices.* However, information alone is not going to make you healthier. It is up to you to put *your* smart choices into action, not just today, but every day. We want you to be informed, motivated—and above all healthy!

Reed V. Tuckson, MD, FACP
Executive Vice President and
Chief of Medical Affairs, UnitedHealth Group

PART ONE

51 WELLNESS BOOSTERS

Smart Choices Today for a Healthier Tomorrow

EACH DAY BRINGS US A NEW CHANCE TO MAKE SMALL-BUT-smart lifestyle changes that have a big impact on our health. Take a walk after dinner instead of heading to the couch, for example. Spend a few minutes unwinding and letting go of the day's stress. Get caught up on your sleep. Simple choices such as these really do make a difference. In this section, you'll find many more helpful ideas. You'll also get some great tips for making these changes work in your everyday life. So, give your health and well-being a boost today. Start making the healthy changes you've been putting off—and watch the benefits add up.

Eating Well: 11 Essentials

Food is one area where you can really grab control of your health. The average person makes more than 200 food choices each day, beginning with what to have for breakfast. The good news? Each decision is a new chance to eat smarter.

Everything you eat affects your body in a different way. The immediate benefit is taste. But, food also fuels your body and gives you energy. Some foods may help lower your risk of getting diseases, such as certain cancers, diabetes and heart disease. Choosing the right foods most of the time may help some people live a longer, healthier life.

Eating well doesn't demand a complete pantry makeover. Even small steps may help you move closer to better health. So, dig in to these 11 smart choices—intended for most healthy adults—and start making them work for you!

1 ➤ PICK THE RIGHT CARBS

Low-carbohydrate diets are popular. But, the truth is, your body needs carbs. Carbs are converted into a fuel called glucose (blood sugar). It feeds your cells and organs, including your brain. If half your total calories come from carbs, you're within a normal, healthful range.

Carbs are found in pasta, sugar and vegetables. You can probably see right away that some of these foods have more value than others. Try to avoid carbs such as corn syrup and table sugar. They offer only empty calories. There's an easy way to judge whether or not your carbs are worth eating. Smart carb choices fall into at least one of these two groups:

Rich in fiber. Fiber is a part of plant foods that can't be digested. But, it still delivers many benefits. Fiber helps your stomach feel full faster. This may prevent weight gain. It also helps keep things on track in your digestive system by helping prevent constipation. Most important, a high-fiber diet may help lower your risk of diabetes and heart disease. You'll find a lot of fiber in certain fruits and vegetables. Legumes (beans, peas and peanuts) and whole grains are other great sources. Try to get 20 to 35 grams of fiber every day.

Multitaskers. Natural foods such as fruits, vegetables and milk give your body carbs. But, they also give you a host of vitamins and minerals. Choose these multitasking carbs as your main source.

Adding Fiber

Here are some ways to get more fiber in your diet.

- Select whole-grain breads and pastas, and brown rice, instead of white varieties.
- Choose oat and other whole-grain cereals.
- Have a salad every day.
- Sprinkle wheat bran on salads and low- or non-fat yogurt.
- Eat whole fruits instead of juices. Fruit skin, like vegetable skin, is loaded with fiber. Be sure to wash the fruits first.

---

2 ▶ SHIFT TO BETTER FATS

Fats are important because they give you energy. Fats also help your body absorb vitamins. But, every gram of fat has nine calories. Eating too much fat may put you at risk of obesity and heart disease. Here's an easy rule: Twenty to 35 percent of your calories should come from fat. You can find fat and calorie information on nutrition facts labels. The percentages given on these labels are based on a 2,000-calorie diet.

It's important to know that not all fats are created equal. There are six main types. Three of them are seen as risky fats—saturated fat, trans fat and food cholesterol. That's because they may hurt your blood cholesterol levels. The other three are healthful—monounsaturated and polyunsaturated fats, and omega-3 fatty acids. They may help improve your cholesterol levels.

Here are some quick facts that can help you recognize and choose healthful fats:

Fats to Limit or Avoid

- Saturated fat comes from high-fat dairy products, meat, poultry skin, chocolate, and coconut and palm oils. Avoid getting more than 10 percent of your total calories from saturated fat. Do this by limiting yourself to less than 15 grams of saturated fat per day.
- Trans fat is found in stick margarine and shortening. Many packaged snack foods, such as chips, cookies and crackers, often contain trans fat. It's best to avoid these fats.
- Cholesterol in food comes mainly from animal products, such as meats, poultry, shellfish and eggs. Butter, cheese, and whole or 2 percent milk also have cholesterol. Try to limit yourself to fewer than 300 milligrams of cholesterol each day.

Fats to Favor

- Monounsaturated fat comes from nuts, sesame seeds, avocados, and canola and olive oils.
- Polyunsaturated fat is found in soft margarine and some oils, including corn, safflower, soybean and sunflower.
- Omega-3 fatty acids are found in certain fish. This includes salmon, sardines and tuna. It's also in soy products, walnuts and some oils, such as flaxseed.

Trimming the Fat

Swapping full-fat foods for lower-fat versions is a great way to cut calories. For example, 1 cup of regular small-curd cottage cheese has 9 grams of fat (81 fat calories). But, 1 cup of cottage cheese made with 1 percent low-fat milk has only 2 grams of fat (18 fat calories). Check out a few more dietary switches that will help cut calories without losing flavor:

TRY...	INSTEAD OF...
Fat-free or low-fat milk	Whole milk
Baked tortilla chips	Regular potato chips
Light margarine with added plant stanols	Butter
Grilled chicken	Fried chicken
Fat-free frozen yogurt	Ice cream
Reduced-fat cheese	Full-fat cheese
Mustard	Mayonnaise

3 ▶ POWER UP WITH LEAN PROTEIN

Protein is key for building blood, bone, muscle and skin. It gives you essential vitamins and minerals. It helps your immune system, protects your cells and much more. Protein-rich foods include all meats, poultry and fish. Eggs, seeds, nuts and peanut butter also count. Lentils, dry beans and peas, and soybeans (tofu)—known as legumes—are in both the meat and vegetable groups. However, you'll only need to think about counting legumes as meat if you're a vegetarian. See Building Protein, Vegetarian Style, Page 17.

Most adults need five or six meat equivalents every day. About an ounce of meat, poultry or fish equals one meat equivalent. Here's a rundown of your protein choices:

Meats

Some meats are high in saturated fat and cholesterol. This may raise your blood cholesterol and lead to heart disease. So, it's important to make smart choices in this area. This doesn't mean you should never eat meat. Instead, be aware of options that are more healthful and how much you're eating. Beef, lamb and pork have the most saturated fat. Avoid fatty cuts. Also, look for alternatives to regular ground beef, bacon, bologna, sausage and the like. Many are available in low-fat or poultry versions. These may be more healthful choices. Check the labels to find out.

When cooking, try using only half of the meat called for in a recipe. Substitute beans or lentils for the other half. Or, serve a small amount of meat as a side dish. And, serve the leanest choices. This includes ground beef that's labeled *lean* or *extra-lean* (90 percent to 95 percent lean). Other lean choices are sirloin, loin, round or chuck cuts of beef, in "choice" or "select" grades. Lamb cuts from the loin or leg, and pork tenderloin and loin chops are also good.

Be sure to cook all meats thoroughly before serving.

Poultry

Chicken, turkey and duck make up the poultry group. The white meat from chicken and turkey is very heart-healthful. But, be sure to remove the skin. Duck is higher in saturated fat. Eat this only occasionally.

Fish

Fatty fish, such as salmon, mackerel and herring, have omega-3 fatty acids. That's one of the heart-healthful fats. Experts recommend eating fish at least two times a week.

Fish Advisory for Pregnant Women

Fish is an important part of a healthful diet. If you're a woman who's pregnant or nursing or who may become pregnant, choose low-mercury fish, such as canned light tuna, catfish, pollack, salmon and shrimp. Don't eat king mackerel, shark, swordfish or tilefish. They all contain high levels of mercury. Keep your total fish intake to no more than 12 ounces per week of low-mercury fish.

Eggs

Eggs count as part of your daily meat-equivalent limit. One egg equals one meat. A single egg yolk delivers more than half of your daily allowance of food cholesterol. If your cholesterol is higher than it should be, it's smart to eat no more than four egg yolks per week.

A Smarter Way to Use Eggs

You can cut cholesterol and fat by using only egg whites for your breakfast scramble or omelet. Also, substitute two egg whites for each whole egg in recipes that call for eggs.

Seeds and Nuts

Some seeds and nuts are a good source of healthful fat. But, watch how many you're eating. Just half an ounce of seeds or nuts—roughly a small handful—or a tablespoon of peanut butter count as one meat. Don't forget that some nut products have a high salt content. And, the ingredients of some nut butters include added salt and sugar.

Building Protein, Vegetarian Style

People whose diets don't include meat—or include only small amounts of it—should pay special attention to legumes. A quarter-cup of legumes, such as chickpeas, kidney beans or lentils, counts as one meat equivalent. This means it has the same amount of dietary protein. A quarter cup of tofu or 2 tablespoons of hummus also counts as one meat equivalent.

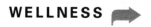

4 MIND YOUR VITAMINS AND MINERALS

More than two dozen essential vitamins and minerals are high on the list of what your body needs from food. For example, they help build and maintain bone strength. They also activate white blood cells and control infections. On the opposite page, you'll find an at-a-glance guide to some of these vital nutrients.

5 ELIMINATE EXTRA SODIUM

Sodium helps our muscles and nerves work. But, a little goes a long way. If your doctor hasn't limited your sodium intake, you can have about 2,300 milligrams daily. You won't have to work hard to reach this level. It's about the size of a teaspoon of table salt. The average American takes in 2,900 to 4,300 milligrams of sodium every day. That's alarming when you consider that for some people, eating too much sodium may lead to high blood pressure and a greater risk of stroke.

But, it's easy to consume too much sodium. It's found in so many processed foods, including condiments. It's also a flavor booster that many of us like to use when cooking and eating. Try using salt alternatives, such as spices, to help reduce sodium intake. Also, try using dried and fresh fruits and berries or flavored vinegars in your cooking. They're a tasty way to liven up your meals.

Doing the Numbers

Your body needs several essential nutrients. That's where daily values (DVs) come in. DVs are used on food labels so that you know the basic nutrient content of what you're eating. They're not recommended intakes. But, they do tell you the percentage of the daily value of each nutrient in a serving of the food.

Nutrient	May Help This Way	Where to Find It	Recommended 2008 Daily Intake (RDI) for Adults*
Calcium	Makes and preserves bone; helps with nerve impulses; helps in heart rhythm	Milk, cheese and yogurt; broccoli and kale; fortified cereals and fruit juices	1,000 mg through age 50; 1,200 mg for ages 51 and older
Magnesium	Assists with muscle functioning and heart rhythm; helps immune system; strengthens bones	Legumes; whole grains; seeds and nuts; spinach	310 mg for women; 400 mg for men
Potassium	Contributes to blood pressure control; assists in organ, tissue and cell functioning	Salmon, flounder and cod; chicken; soy products; sweet potatoes and lima beans; bananas; oranges; milk products; most fruits and vegetables	4.7 gm
Vitamin A (retinol or beta carotene)	Assists with immune system functioning; assists with bone strength	Milk products; fortified cereals; orange vegetables	700 mcg of retinol for women; 900 mcg of retinol for men
B Vitamins (folate, B-6 and B-12)	Helps prevent neurological damage and neurological birth defects	Fortified cereals; fruits; vegetables; legumes; whole grains; milk products; fish; poultry	400 mcg of folate; 1.3–1.7 mg of B-6; 2.4 mcg of B-12
Vitamin C	May protect against free radicals, which damage cells and cause diseases	Citrus fruits; tomatoes; spinach and peppers; fortified cereals	75 mg for women; 90 mg for men
Vitamin D	Boosts bone health; may guard against some cancers	Salmon and tuna; fortified cereals and fruit juice; milk and milk products	400–800 international units (IU)

*RDIs are for healthy adults. Pregnant or nursing women should check with their doctors.

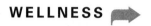

6 ▸ DRINK WATER FOR GOOD HEALTH

Water is important to your health. It helps move nutrients to your cells and organs. It also may be a great tool for weight management, especially if you drink water instead of sugary drinks. After all, water contains no calories or fat. These tips may help you get your fill:

Let your thirst guide you. Most healthy individuals will get enough fluids by simply drinking water during meals and, of course, whenever thirsty. Speaking of thirst, plain old water remains the drink of choice to quench it.

Zest it up. If you don't like the taste of plain water, try adding a lemon, lime or cucumber slice.

7 ▸ GO FOR WHOLE GRAINS

Grains are plant foods made from barley, corn, oats, rice and more. As with fats, some grains are better than others. Grains processed with the outer coat and heart of the grain intact are called whole grains. They're better for you than refined grains. That's because refined grains have been stripped of their essential fiber, vitamins and minerals. Eating whole grains has been tied to a number of health benefits. Increased longevity is one. Reduced risk of heart disease and better weight control are others. Whole grains should make up at least half of the grains you eat every day. That's about three servings (or ounce equivalents) for most people.

A peek inside most kitchen pantries would probably reveal a lot of refined grains, such as white bread and white rice. But, it's easy to replace those with more healthful, whole-grain options. On the next page, you'll find a list of whole grains that may help you make more healthful—and tasty—diet choices.

Barley. This grain may help control your cholesterol. Look for hulled or hull-less barley.

Corn. Choices include whole corn, whole-grain cornmeal and popcorn.

Oats. Oats are known for their cholesterol-lowering ability. They're most often found in breakfast cereals. Check the ingredients to be sure *"whole oats"* is listed. Steel-cut oats are often found in oatmeal. They're whole-grain oats that have been cut, not rolled, for a more dense texture.

Quinoa. Try it as a light side dish.

Brown rice. This alternative to white rice is a good whole-grain choice.

Whole wheat. It's the most popular grain in America. Try whole-wheat pasta and bread.

Other whole grains. Buckwheat, bulgur wheat, rye and wheat berries are just a few of the many other varieties.

8 ADD COLORFUL VEGETABLES

You already know that vegetables contain a wide range of vitamins and minerals. They're also a fiber-rich source of carbs. Cooked, raw, dried, canned, frozen or even in juice, vegetables of all varieties can have a big impact on your health. Eating them may lower your risk of heart disease, stroke, Type 2 diabetes, certain cancers and more. Most people should eat 2½ to 3 cups of vegetables every day. That's about 3 servings.

But, don't get stuck in a veggie rut. Different vegetables offer different nutrients. For example, orange vegetables are an excellent source of beta-carotene. So reach for those carrots, squashes and sweet potatoes.

Dark-green vegetables, such as broccoli, collard greens and leafy green lettuces, are also bursting with nutrients. Corn, green peas and potatoes—known as starchy vegetables—have a lot to offer as well. So do legumes, such as chickpeas, kidney beans, lentils, soybeans, split peas and white beans. Looking for time-saving and delicious ways to eat more vegetables? Try these ideas:

Rely on ready-to-eat. Buy fresh vegetables that are already cut and washed. Or, try one of the many frozen vegetables that come ready to steam in the microwave.

Liven up salads. Try Boston, green-leaf, red-leaf or romaine lettuces. Or, toss in some spinach leaves. Add chopped veggies that are outside your normal fare, such as whole peas in the pod and zucchini. Also, fruits such as red grapes or avocados make good salad additions. Drizzle with a bit of flavored vinegar.

Experiment. Try making veggies in new ways. You might not like cooked spinach, for example, but you might love it raw in a salad. Flavorings such as garlic can liven up a sautéed or grilled vegetable dish. Try adding pureed vegetables to sauces, soups and stews. Or, add chopped vegetables to casseroles, lasagna and muffins.

9 ▸ GET YOUR FILL OF FRUITS

Eating a wide variety of fruits has many benefits. High-fruit diets may help lower rates of heart disease, stroke, Type 2 diabetes, certain cancers and more. Fruits have no cholesterol. But, they may help *control* yours. And, they're generally low in fat, calories and sodium. Aim for at least 1½ to 2 cups of fruit every day. That's about 2 servings. Here are some of the superstars to know:

Dark-colored fruits. These often owe their coloring to anthocyanin, which is linked to a lower risk of cancer. Find it in blackberries, blueberries, plums, tart cherries and even green kiwi.

Light red and pink fruits. Guava, tomatoes, watermelon, and pink and red grapefruits contain lycopene. Researchers are looking into lycopene for its possible role in heart disease and cancer prevention.

Red grapes. These contain high levels of resveratrol, which is linked to the prevention of cancer and heart disease. Other research suggests it also may help lower the risk of Alzheimer's disease.

Counting Calories

Follow these steps to learn how many calories you should eat in order to lose weight:

1. Multiply your weight by 10 to get your base calories.
2. Multiply your weight by three if you're sedentary, by five if you're moderately active, or by eight if you're very active. This number represents your activity calories.
3. Add your base calories and activity calories. The total is the number of calories you'd need to eat to maintain your current weight. If you're older than age 50, subtract 10 percent of this number for your adjusted calorie count.
4. Eat 500 fewer calories per day. You should lose a pound a week. If you cut down by 1,000 calories per day, you should lose about 2 pounds per week. Keep in mind that weight loss rates vary by individual. Ask your doctor about a safe minimum calorie intake for your needs and lifestyle.

10 ▶ MILK THE BENEFITS

Milk and most milk products are packed with calcium, potassium and added vitamin D. These nutrients help make and keep bones strong. They may also help prevent osteoporosis and control your blood pressure. Most adults should have 3 cups of milk or milk products daily.

Like milk, other milk products usually range in fat content from fat-free to 1 percent, 2 percent and whole (full fat). Consuming full-fat milk or milk products on a regular basis may hurt your blood cholesterol levels. It may also increase your risk of heart disease. Choose fat-free and low-fat instead. Switching from whole milk to fat-free will save you more than 65 calories per 1-cup serving.

Here are ways to work low-fat calcium into your diet:
• Stock up on fat-free or low-fat string cheese.
• Drink a serving-size carton of fat-free chocolate milk.
• Grab a single-serve container of fat-free or low-fat yogurt.
• Enjoy a snack size of low-fat pudding.

11 ▶ MAINTAIN A HEALTHFUL WEIGHT

When it comes to losing weight if you're overweight or obese, small steps mean a lot. In fact, losing as little as 5 percent of your weight may lead to significant health benefits. These include better blood cholesterol and blood pressure levels. You'll also lower your risk of heart disease and Type 2 diabetes. So, the first important step in coming up with a weight loss plan is setting reasonable goals.

Here are a few tips to help you get started:

Talk with your doctor. Check with your doctor about the best weight range for you. Discuss how to get there safely. Talk about an appropriate exercise plan. If you've been unsuccessful at weight management in the past, ask for a referral to a registered dietitian.

Eat fewer calories than you burn. Everyone's calorie needs are different. So, your calorie plan for losing weight should be customized, too. See Counting Calories, Page 24, for a general guideline.

Lose at a safe rate. Losing about one-half to 2 pounds a week is best for most people. Losing more than that may make your new eating patterns difficult to keep up for any length of time. This could cause you to regain the weight down the road. Only take part in an aggressive weight-loss plan under the guidance of your doctor.

Eat smart. Traditionally, losing weight has meant eating less. But, research shows you don't necessarily have to eat less to lose weight. You just have to eat foods with fewer calories. That means eating smarter. For example, try making pasta casseroles with less pasta and meat and more vegetables.

Aim for balance. The most complete and helpful guide to balancing your diet is the U.S. Department of Agriculture's Food Guide Pyramid. It's customizable based on your age, gender, weight, height and level of activity. See MyPyramid for Food Choices, Page 228.

Switching Gears

Eating smart doesn't have to mean eating bland. The next time you're craving a traditional favorite, try the following switches. They may help cut calories *and* boost nutrition:

- Veggie pizza on a whole-wheat crust topped with a light sprinkle of low-fat mozzarella cheese.
- Half-serving of cereal topped with fresh fruit and fat-free milk.
- Salad topped with a cup of chopped grilled chicken.
- One egg (instead of two) scrambled with your favorite vegetables.
- Low-fat chicken broth made with a cup of chopped vegetables, some legumes and brown rice. Skip the meat.
- Grill, sauté, roast, steam, broil, stir-fry or bake instead frying.
- For low-calorie snack choices, check out 10 Snacks Under 100 Calories, Page 231.

Get Active: 7 Ideas That Work

Staying active is one of the best things you can do for your health. Regular exercise directly affects the strength of your bones and some of your body's most important muscles, including your heart. Doing some form of exercise every day may reduce your risk of heart disease, stroke, osteoporosis and diabetes. It also may help lower your cholesterol and blood pressure, and help prevent obesity. More energy and a better metabolism are other pluses. Exercise may even help you handle stress.

Look for ways to make physical activity part of your everyday lifestyle. For some, this might mean going to the local gym. For others, it could mean making changes such as taking the stairs instead of the elevator. Or, taking a walk after dinner might become a new routine. What matters is that you're moving your body. Because when you move, you're helping your heart and lungs to work better. You're also building flexibility and strength.

Boosting your activity level is a great idea. But, be certain to check with your doctor before starting *any* exercise program. This includes stretching and strength training. And, take a look at the guidelines for building more activity into your routine that are included in this chapter.

12 ▸ PLAY IT SAFE

Once you've decided to get active, it's tempting to try to make up for lost time. But, the best approach is to start slowly. Build up the intensity and length of your exercise gradually. Check in with your doctor. He or she may be able to suggest a workout plan that's right for your lifestyle.

Next, learn how to track your heart rate. Monitor how you're doing by keeping tabs on your pulse during your workouts. With one or two fingers (not your thumb), lightly touch one of the large blood vessels on your neck, beside your Adam's apple. Or, take your pulse on the inside of your wrist, closer to your thumb. Count the number of beats in 10 seconds. Multiply this number by six. That gives you an approximate number of beats per minute (bpm). Ideally, this number should fall within your target heart rate zone (see the chart below). If you're younger than age 25 or older than age 65, ask your doctor if these bpm ranges apply to you.

Another important number is your maximum heart rate. Simply subtract your age from 220. The answer is your maximum heart rate. During exercise, your goal should be to keep your heart rate between 50 percent to 85 percent of your maximum. This range is commonly called your target heart rate zone. Beginners should aim for the lower end of the scale. Then, they can slowly build toward 85 percent. Over time, checking your heart rate will help you keep track of your fitness level and progress.

Age	Average Maximum Heart Rate	Target Zone: 50%–85% of maximum
25	195	98–166
30	190	95–162
35	185	93–157
40	180	90–153
45	175	88–149
50	170	85–145
55	165	83–140
60	160	80–136
65	155	78–132

Source: Centers for Disease Control and Prevention

Note: If you take medicine to control high blood pressure, be aware that some drugs lower the maximum heart rate. Ask your doctor if you also should lower your target heart rate.

13   INCLUDE AEROBIC WORKOUTS

Aerobic activities make you breathe deeply and get your blood pumping for an extended period of time. They give your heart, lungs and other muscles a workout. You may even feel like you have more energy. These heart-pumping workouts also help reduce stress and prevent heart disease, diabetes, stroke and some cancers. So, it's important that your exercise routine includes some type of aerobic activity.

Traditional aerobic activities are walking, running, step aerobics, biking, hiking, swimming and skiing. But, dancing and everyday activities such as walking up the stairs are, too. Try to build aerobic workouts into your schedule most days of the week. For the best results, do them for at least 30 minutes over the course of the day. Here are a few ideas:

Just walk. Walking is a great calorie burner—as long as you walk fast. Walking is also a weight-bearing activity. That means you hold your weight and work against gravity in order to do it. Weight-bearing activities strengthen your bones and help prevent osteoporosis. And, it's so easy. Just grab a good pair of walking shoes and go.

Dive in. Swimming is a no-sweat aerobic activity that's also gentle on your joints. If swimming's your main aerobic activity, try varying your strokes and speed. This way you'll work more muscles. And, you'll have more fun. Just remember, it's not a weight-bearing exercise. So, it can't help protect your bones.

Work out at home. Home equipment, such as stationary bikes, treadmills and fitness DVDs, makes aerobic exercise convenient. Keep the equipment in plain sight. That way, you'll be more likely to use it.

Follow the fun. Join a sports league or take dance lessons. Choose an aerobic activity that you'll enjoy. After all, the best exercise is something you'll want to stick with.

Rehydrate After a Workout

Energy drinks may be high in sugar. And, they may only be beneficial if your aerobic workouts go beyond 45 minutes. For most people, water is the best thirst quencher.

---

14 ▶ BUILD STRENGTH

Strength training—also known as resistance training or weight lifting—refers to working the muscles in your body. This builds strong muscles and bones. The goal isn't to look like Mr. Universe. In fact, anyone can benefit from strength training. But, be sure to check with your doctor first.

Even the smallest amount of training may improve and balance your core. These are the muscles in your abdomen and middle back. Strength training may also help keep your weight in check by increasing metabolism. And, it may help prevent osteoporosis. Strength training can be done using free weights or weight-training machines. You can even skip the gym and do calisthenics, such as push-ups. Here are a few tips for getting started:

Know your zone. The key to strength training is staying in your comfort zone. Recognize your limits. There's no shame in starting with 1- to 2-pound weights. Gradually add more weight to push yourself. Remember that strength-training workouts are meant to challenge your muscles. So, if you can't do eight to 10 repetitions, you're probably using too much weight.

Move smoothly and slowly. For example, take three seconds to do a full lift. Hold it for one second. Then release for three more seconds. Don't forget to breathe! Start big. First, work your larger muscles—your thighs, back, chest and abdominals. Then move on to the smaller ones, such as your arms and calves.

Don't forget to rest. Overworked muscles may cause muscle exhaustion and strain. It could also lead to injury. Never target the same muscle groups two days in a row or more than three times a week.

Adding Strength

Here are four ways to add strength training to your regular routine:

1. Bring in bags of groceries or firewood.
2. Carry a small child (under 25 pounds).
3. Mow the lawn with a push mower.
4. Put out full bags of trash and recyclables.

---

15 ▶ STAY FLEXIBLE

Including a flexibility program in your exercise routine is an important part of staying active. It can help improve joint range of motion and joint flexibility. This can allow for moving more easily, better balance and less pain in your joints. You can try yoga or tai chi. Doing some easy stretches throughout the day is another good option.

Taking the Extra Step

Here are five ways you can work light activity into your day:

1. Take stretch breaks.
2. Garden.
3. Climb stairs.
4. Swing your child or grandchild at the playground.
5. Walk whenever you can.

General Exercise Tips

It's a good idea to ease into and out of any exercise routine. Here are some simple tips:

WARM UP. Warm up your muscles for five to 10 minutes before you exercise. Start with an endurance exercise you can do at low speed, such as walking instead of running. Gentle limb movements are great warm-ups. Try twisting your torso slowly from side to side. Then, make large swooping motions with your arms. And, lift your knees one at a time. Be careful not to stretch or move to the point of pain.

COOL DOWN. Taking five to 10 minutes to cool your body down after exercise is important, too. It may be easiest to repeat your warm-up routine. Or, try slowing down your workout activity to a minimal level. This slows your heart rate. At the same time, gently stretch your muscles.

---

16 ▸ EXERCISE FOR WEIGHT CONTROL

Movement is more than a key part of healthful living. It's also a vital part of a successful weight-control program. That's because you have to burn more calories than you consume to lose weight. You won't achieve this without exercise.

The key to success is sticking with your exercise routine. This is true whether you're someone for whom pounds melt away almost effortlessly or you have to work extra hard. For weight loss, a good rule of thumb is to aim for 60 minutes of moderately intense physical activity on most days of the week.

If you're not sure whether you need to lose weight, talk with your doctor. He or she also may provide advice on the best exercise program for you. For a quick estimate using your height and weight, see Your Healthful Weight, Page 226.

17 ▸ JOIN THE RIGHT GYM FOR YOU

While certainly not necessary, a gym membership can open up a world of new experiences. You'll discover new workout equipment and classes. Fitness professionals trained to help you also will be on hand. These tips can help you find a gym that's right for you:

Shop around. Ask about trial memberships at various gyms. Take tours and ask questions about how the equipment works. Sit in on classes and programs to decide if what they offer appeals to you.

Ask about fitness assessments. You should be offered not only an initial health assessment, but also regular screenings to gauge your improvement.

Be safe. Look for a clean, well-maintained, well-staffed and well-lit gym. Emergency equipment, including an automatic heart defibrillator, should be in place. Most important, the staff should know how to use all of this equipment.

Seek qualifications. Professional gym staff should be knowledgeable about exercise science. They should hold exercise certifications through a reputable organization. The American College of Sports Medicine is a good example.

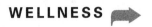

Going for the Gusto

Try these five ways to add more moderate activity to your day:

1. Take your dog for a walk.
2. Dance—any music, any style.
3. Turn off the TV and take a walk around the block or local mall.
4. Hand wash your car.
5. Park your car away from any entrance and walk.

For more ideas, see Calories Burned During Activities, Page 231.

---

18 ▶ ## STAY MOTIVATED

You may think exercise is going to be too hard. That you have too many pounds to lose. That it just won't work. Or, that you just shouldn't try. But, it *will* work if you stick with it. Physical activity is a gift that keeps giving. With each week of committed exercise, you'll grow stronger in small but meaningful ways. Before you know it, it won't take a lot of effort to do your daily activities. Keep your motivation strong by trying these tips:

Book it. Put notes on your refrigerator to remind yourself of your fitness dates. Add them to your calendar. This will help you commit to your activities and stay on track.

Make the time fly. Ride an exercise bike while listening to a book on tape or watching your favorite TV show.

Wake up your walks. Go somewhere special on your next walk. Some ideas? Walk around a zoo or a museum. Or, walk around a neighborhood of unique homes. Keep your pace brisk.

Get a buddy boost. Find someone to do your activities with. You'll be able to enjoy some social time while you work out. And, don't forget the family pet. Your dog may make a great walking or jogging partner.

Make it an adventure. Mix up your exercise routine by trying new activities, with new people and in new settings. If you always work out indoors, go outside, and vice versa.

Remember the benefits. Make a list of what exercise may do for you. Here's one to get you started: You may be able to lower your blood pressure with as little as three to four weeks of regular exercise. Add to the list anything that gets you inspired—from clothes that fit better to having more energy.

Reward yourself for meeting goals. For example, treat yourself to a movie night for getting through two full weeks of workouts.

The Best Motivator of All—Better Health

Don't let yourself be a couch potato. Get up and move, however you can. Remember, you can improve your quality of life with as little as 10 to 30 minutes of exercise every day.

Less Stress! 4 Secrets of Positive Living

Your chances of living a long, healthy life depend on more than good genes and luck. How we cope with life's everyday challenges also plays a big role.

More and more, research shows that a positive outlook is good for our health. Being optimistic lowers the risk of disease. Happier people tend to have lower rates of high blood pressure. They also may have better memories and a stronger immune system.

But, what if you're not naturally a happy-go-lucky person? There's hope. We all have the power to change how we react to life's ups and downs—and to stress.

Stress is a part of life. But, it can be your friend or enemy. It may spark you to get out of bed bright and early to get a jump-start on your busy day. Or, it may make you feel like the weight of the world is on your shoulders.

Over time, stress may take a real toll, both on your body and your spirit. During times of stress, your body makes high levels of the hormones adrenaline and cortisol. These stress hormones do several things once released. They can cause your heart rate to go up, for example. These hormones also cause your breathing to accelerate and your blood vessels to narrow. These changes can protect and help you if you need to respond quickly to a threat. However, if this response occurs too often, it can be damaging. It may lead to fatigue, heart disease, high blood pressure, obesity and other health problems.

For all of these reasons, learning to take things in stride is important to your health. The good news is that little things go a long way when it comes to lowering your stress. But, no single approach works for everyone. So, it's good to try a few different techniques. Then, you see which works best for you.

19 ▶ BE AWARE

Before you can get a handle on stress, you first need to understand how it affects you. Then, you need to be able to recognize what sets off your stress responses. Here are some things to consider:

Know the signs. How do you feel when you're stressed out? You might get anxious, irritable or depressed. You may want to cry. Your muscles may tense up. Or, you may have a hard time sleeping. Keep in mind, these symptoms may also be caused by certain medical conditions, not just stress. If you're having any of the above symptoms for several days, call your doctor.

Note the triggers. Once you pinpoint your signs of stress, look for the causes. When your jaw clenches shut or your head begins to pound, what's going on in your life? Maybe you had a fight with a friend. Or, you got an unexpected bill. Anything from being sick to having a rough patch at work can send stress hormones racing. Write down specific things that push your stress buttons.

Take charge of your reactions. Try to avoid turning to cigarettes, food or alcohol to make you feel better. In the long run, these behaviors may cause even more stress. They may even cause health problems. You may find yourself in the difficult spot of having to quit smoking, lose weight or cope with a drinking problem. Explore positive ways to respond to stress. Take the time to put these new responses into practice. Your health and peace of mind will benefit.

> ## Going Gray?
> **There is no proven link between stress and gray hair. Hair turns gray when cells stop producing the color pigment melanin. This happens naturally as we age.**

20 ▶ LEARN TO RELAX

Here are some ways to help you relax and regain control of your emotions:

Exercise. One of the best ways to relieve stress is to get moving for 30 to 60 minutes a day, most days of the week. See the Get Active chapter, Page 27, for lots of ideas. A fit body is more prepared to cope with stress than an unfit one. And, exercise is known to boost your overall well-being. Be sure to talk with your doctor before beginning any new exercise program.

Do something you enjoy. Fun is another powerful tool for showing stress the door. When you're doing something you enjoy, it's hard to remain stressed-out. Listen to music, read a book or get a pedicure. Making time for things you enjoy is just as important as running errands and paying bills.

Learn a new trick. You can train your body to respond to stress differently. Try taking a few moments each day to relax all the muscles in your body. Start by taking a few deep breaths. Then, relax the muscles in your head and face. Don't forget your jaw muscles. They tighten when you're stressed. Next, relax your shoulders. Let your arms drop to your sides. Rest your hands on top of your thighs. Finally, relax all the muscles in your legs and feet.

Eat smart. Eating lots of fresh fruits and vegetables, whole grains, and lean protein will make it easier to fight the bad effects of stress. For more tips, see Eating Well, Page 12.

21   **GET RID OF ANGER**

Everything that happens to you throughout the course of the day, from getting a parking ticket to not having enough change for a snack, sparks a mental response. If you find yourself thinking, "Here we go again," or "This is just my luck," you're going to feel stressed. Instead, try to keep things in perspective. While we can't always control the situation, we can control how we respond.

Anger is a basic human emotion. But, high levels of anger can affect your health, your work and your relationships. When you're angry, your body naturally produces more of the hormone adrenaline. This gives you the energy to take action. But, too much of it may lead to health problems. People who are often angry have a higher risk of heart disease and heart attacks, compared to those who keep their cool.

If you have a tendency to get too angry, chances are you know it. Acting out of control or in a way that frightens others are two signs that it's probably time to find new ways to handle life's upsets. However, some people with an anger problem may actually withdraw from others. Or, they often feel testy and cranky, but may not act on it. Trying to bottle things up isn't good either.

If your anger or frustration is spilling over into your personal or work life, consider talking with a licensed mental health professional. Many workplaces offer programs that can connect you with helpful resources. Ask your human resources department.

These tips can help those who want to rein in their anger:

Give yourself a timeout. Getting hot under the collar? Find a spot where you can be alone and cool off. Take some deep breaths to help relax your speeding heart rate and rising adrenaline level. You also may find it helpful to do this at a set time every day. For example, take a few minutes after work to simply do nothing. Then, tackle the mail, dinner or other priorities.

Practice relaxation techniques. Deep breathing is one great way to lessen your anger. The right way to breathe is from deep in your gut, not from your chest. Visualization is another way to relax. Close your eyes. Think of a time or place in your life when you were very happy. Regular exercise helps, too. But, check with your doctor first.

Don't sweep anger under the rug. Keeping anger inside may contribute to high blood pressure, depression or other medical conditions. But, it's not beneficial to take your anger out on others by exploding. The most positive way to address anger is to express it in a calm, clear way. Tell the person you're upset with why you're angry. Be careful not to put him on the defensive. Use "I feel" statements, such as, "I feel like I don't have a say." Let him know what your needs are, and what he can do to meet them. Be prepared to listen to his point of view, too.

Retune your thinking. The way you think about a situation may make it worse. If you tell yourself, "This is maddening," you're going to erupt. Instead, speak to yourself in calm, rational terms such as, "This is frustrating, but everything will be all right." Focus on what's within your control.

Think two steps ahead. Try to prepare for situations that stir up your anger. Better yet, avoid them—if possible. For example, if weeknights are busy and hectic, plan to have discussions with your partner on the weekends instead.

22 MANAGE DEPRESSION

Unresolved stress and related anger may increase your risk of depression. Anyone who's experienced this condition knows how crippling it can be. You feel sad, hopeless, helpless and tired. And, you may lose interest in once-loved activities. It's important to know that depression is treatable. The best way to fight it depends on its severity.

Major depression is characterized by a blue mood that lasts for at least two weeks. This sadness gets in the way of everyday activities, such as working, sleeping and eating. Sufferers also lose interest in things that once brought pleasure and enjoyment. Major depression typically is treated with psychotherapy or prescription antidepressants, or both. For mild depression, self-help strategies and lifestyle changes may be helpful. In each case, the first step is to see your health care professional.

Nothing takes the place of medical care, counseling and medications, if needed. But, there are additional beneficial steps you can take. These include:

Awareness. Certain lifestyle factors may cause or increase feelings of depression. These include lack of sleep, poor diet, restricted seasonal light, stress, alcohol abuse and relationship problems. Once you recognize the triggers, try changing those that are within your control. Bring the others to the attention of your health care professional.

Exercise. Not only does exercise help you get in shape and tone your muscles, it also raises the amount of feel-good chemicals in the brain. Exercising for at least 30 minutes a day most days of the week is a good approach. Check with your doctor before starting any exercise program.

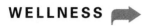
Omega-3s. In addition to their brain and heart benefits, omega-3 fatty acids appear to help mood disorders and depression. The best sources of omega-3s are fatty fish such as herring, mackerel and salmon. Aim for two servings of fatty fish per week. Or, ask your doctor about fish-oil supplements. If you're pregnant, ask your doctor about the safest types of fish to eat. See also, Fish Advisory for Pregnant Women, Page 16.

Supporting Roles

Studies have shown that people with a larger circle of friends tend to live longer than those with fewer social connections. Supportive friends and family members give you an outlet to talk about the things that are stressing you out. They also may offer to help lighten the load. If you're not comfortable talking with friends or family members about your problems, consider talking with a counselor or a member of the clergy. Or, think about getting a pet. Studies link pet ownership with longer life spans. And, pets are great stress relievers for their owners. For more on making good connections, see the next chapter.

7 Ways to Make Healthful Connections

There's no question that eating well, getting plenty of exercise and managing stress are part of the recipe for long-term health. But, there's another key ingredient. It's what researchers call *connectedness*. The emotional ties you have with others support your well-being. In fact, *not* staying connected may put you at a greater risk of health problems, such as high blood pressure and depression.

In terms of what's important in your life, your family and friends are probably already at the top of the list. But, you may not realize how much a good marriage or love relationship, close friends or even a beloved pet may add to better health. What follows are simple ways to build and strengthen your personal connections.

23 ▶ STRENGTHEN LOVE'S BONDS

A long-lasting love may offer much more than the promise of happily ever after. Research has shown that married couples live longer and are healthier than single people. They're less likely to smoke or drink heavily. Married couples also are less likely to suffer from back pain, headaches or other serious conditions. And, they're *more* likely to be physically active.

But, you don't have to be married to get the benefits of a happy partnership. To strengthen the bond between you and your partner, try these tips:

Be a good listener. Whether your partner is sharing a story or working through a problem, let him or her talk. Resist the urge to interrupt. Try to see things through his or her eyes. Offer to help find a solution. Take turns and accept that you may have different points of view.

Give praise. Let your loved one know that you value his or her qualities. Accept the fact that you can't change everything about your partner. Find enjoyment in the characteristics you admire.

Say it without words. Be generous with smiles, holding hands, hugs and other signs of love and affection. Practice random acts of kindness. Give a back rub. Make a favorite meal. Or, bring home a surprise gift of flowers or baseball tickets.

Make time for intimacy. Of course, this is a great way to show your love for your partner. But, sex and close physical contact may offer health benefits, too. They may boost immunities to colds and the flu. And, don't forget, sex burns calories.

Get help. Professional counselors can help couples work through problems. They can show you how to use different ways of communicating. When it comes to your sex life, talk openly and honestly with each other about any concerns. Some sexual problems have a medical cause. These include thyroid conditions and abnormal hormone levels, as well as other issues. Don't be shy. Talk with your doctor about your sexual health.

> ### Getting Physical
> Research suggests a link between regular exercise and better, more frequent sex. So, the next time you're about to log onto the Internet, go for a bike ride or take an exercise class instead. Better yet, make a date to work out *with* your partner. Doing so may put you in the mood to reap the rewards ... together. Check with your doctor before starting any exercise program.

24 ▶ CONNECT WITH FRIENDS

Whether you've had a rough day at work, a long illness or a major loss, good friends often can help you through tough times. They also may be a good influence on health choices. And, friendships help protect against heart disease, obesity, stress and depression.

Each friend has something different to offer. You likely won't be able to share your secret hopes and fears with all of your friends. But, it's important to have at least one person with whom you can open up about your dreams *and* problems. It's also nice to feel understood and appreciated. Feeling comfortable "being yourself" around friends is also important.

If your friendships aren't as strong as you'd like, take heart. With a little work, it's possible to rediscover the things that first brought you together. Here are some other ideas to help you keep close ties:

Revisit your past. Pick up the phone and call an old friend. If you've lost touch, try searching online. Don't worry about what to say. Start by letting him know you've been thinking of him.

Send e-mail. But, don't let it replace face-to-face contact altogether. Use e-mail to stay up-to-date with one another. If distance is a factor, pick up the phone for a chat from time to time.

Schedule visits and plan activities. Plan weekly or monthly get-togethers with a few of your favorite people. A set routine and agreed-upon meeting place make it easier to stay in touch.

When You Don't See Eye to Eye

Disagreements are bound to happen in any relationship. It's how you handle them that matters most. When something upsets you, don't hide it or hold it in. These problems may cause hostility, depression and anger. All of these are risk factors for heart disease. So, be open and honest. Explain why you're angry. Talk about how you think the situation might be improved. Avoid name-calling or blaming.

---

25 ▶ MAKE NEW FRIENDS

If your social circle seems to be getting smaller, you're not alone. According to the American Sociological Association, the average American adult's number of close friends has shrunk by one-third during the last 19 years. Experts say that longer work hours is one likely cause. Our many, many tech gadgets is another. Both make it harder to make and keep close ties. That's because they rob you of valuable face-to-face time with loved ones.

Sure, building new friendships takes work. But, it's worth it. Both in terms of happiness and overall health. New friends may help you get out of a rut. Or, they may spark new ideas and activities. They also may open up a brand new social network. Put these ideas for making new friends to work for you:

Try something new. Sign up for that art class you've always wanted to take. Or, join a chess, bridge or book club.

Try a new perspective. Get to know the people you meet during your everyday life. Make friends with that person you know from the health club, for example. Or, strike up a conversation with people at your place of worship.

Branch out. Try mastering the fine art of small talk. That person you see on the bus every morning may share your love of gardening. Or, your son's soccer coach may be looking for a workout partner. By planting seeds with a little conversation, you may find yourself harvesting a new friend or two.

The Many Faces of Friendship

It's not always your oldest childhood pal who will provide long-term health benefits. The healing power of friendship comes in many forms. Same-stage friends are those who are going through similar experiences as you. For example, you both may be managing chronic illnesses or parenting children who are the same age. Workout friends can be lifesavers. And, the buddy system is a great way to boost your chances of sticking with an exercise routine. Finally, having friends who are much younger or older than you may bring refreshing points of view and very special bonds.

26 BUILD COMMUNITY TIES

Being part of a larger community—civic, spiritual or recreational—may boost both happiness and well-being. People with strong group ties have better mental health and fewer sick days. They also have stronger immune systems.

Whatever you do, if you participate in activities you enjoy, you're more likely to get a lift in mood. You'll also have a better quality of life. To strengthen your group ties, try these ideas:

Get involved. Find something you're passionate about. Then, look for ways to play a role. Check out the local food bank. Coach a kids' soccer team. Or, get involved in a political party, theater group or town project.

Keep learning. Take up a new sport or hobby. Learn how to ski, paint or knit. Take classes at the local college. Sit in on a reading by your favorite author. Following your natural curiosity is a great way to find groups that share your interests.

Be a social butterfly. Go for walks around your neighborhood. Introduce yourself to people. Become a regular at your local coffeehouse or recreation center. Host or help organize a block party.

27 ▶ LIVE IN THE MOMENT

Even the simplest rituals may impact your well-being. Try taking time out of your busy day to do a crossword puzzle. Read the comics. Listen to a beautiful piece of music. Or, simply spend 10 whole minutes in complete silence.

Minding the Body

Yoga's emphasis on the mind-body connection is known to deliver emotional benefits. The discipline has been around for more than 5,000 years. Today, more than 15.2 million Americans practice yoga. Half of those took it up for health reasons. Yoga is known to help lower the body's reaction to stress and tension. It also lowers blood pressure. In addition, it helps increase flexibility, strength and balance.

Source: National Center for Complementary and Alternative Medicine

FEED YOUR SPIRIT

Religious and spiritual activities also can bolster feelings of belonging. But, when it comes to spirituality, one size does not fit all. For some, the connection to a higher power is a priority. Others find satisfaction in philosophies and practices that give meaning or purpose to life. Communing with nature is one example of this. But, in every case, the guiding principle is the same. Spiritual pursuits may provide meaning, hope and inner peace. At the same time, they may support your health and happiness.

If you're not already involved in a spiritual pursuit, take the time to explore what feels right to you. Faith-based communities are found in places of worship. Prayer, ceremonies and other customs may help people cope with stress and crises. Other practices emphasize a mind-body connection. Yoga and meditation are two examples. These practices may help you learn to control your inner thoughts and adjust your perspective. Meditation, in particular, appears to slow down the body's fight-or-flight response to stress. This is the mechanism that causes your heart rate to go up, your breathing to accelerate and your blood vessels to narrow.

Giving Back

Studies show that older adults who volunteer as little as two hours a week may live longer. They also suffer less depression and report fewer incidents of bad health than those who volunteer less often.

Sources: Research on Aging, Journal of Health and Social Behavior

---

29 ➤ TAKE THE PET PRESCRIPTION

If you're a pet owner, you know the joy animals can bring to our lives. Pets provide us with faithful companionship. Now, research shows they also may provide a host of health benefits, such as decreases in blood pressure, cholesterol, triglycerides, stress and feelings of loneliness. Pets also are associated with increased activity, social interaction and overall sense of well-being.

Harness this healing pet power. Start by spending more time with your pet each day. Depending on your pet's needs, make a point of playing with or grooming it. Take your dog for long walks as often as possible. If you don't have a pet, think about borrowing one. You could offer to do the dog-walking for a busy neighbor, for example. Or, volunteer at an animal shelter. According to experts, you'll experience health benefits by spending just 30 minutes a day taking a dog for a walk.

Your Doctor & You: 9 Ways to Build a Strong Relationship

Many people only visit their doctors when they're sick. But, seeing your doctor when you're feeling fine makes a lot of sense, too. In fact, having a strong, ongoing relationship with a primary care doctor may make a world of difference to your health.

People who take an active part in their own health care are often happier with the care they get than those who aren't as involved. How can you be one of those satisfied health care consumers? Working closely with a doctor you trust is a great place to start.

30 ▶ CHOOSE A DOCTOR

The first step is to choose a primary care doctor. You may want to ask family and friends for some names. Be sure to check your health plan's list of network doctors. Using doctors who aren't in the network means you'll have to pay more out of your own pocket. And, there are other things to keep in mind. Location, hours, language, even gender, also may be important to you.

Most primary care doctors fall into these three groups:

Family practice doctors. These doctors are trained to provide care, including preventive care, to people of all ages. That means most members of your family can see the same doctor. And, he or she will know your whole family's medical history.

Internists. Adult disease is the area of specialty for these doctors. They focus on prevention and treatment. This can include everything from common ailments to rare illnesses. Some focus broadly on adult medicine. Others also have a sub-specialty in one or more areas.

Geriatric doctors. These doctors focus on the care of older adults. They're trained to look for and address health issues related to aging. They're usually family practice doctors or internists. But, they also have training in geriatric medicine.

Once you have your list of possible primary care doctors, it's a good idea to call each office. Ask questions that will help you decide if the doctor is a good match for you.

Does he or she feel the same way you do about health issues that matter to you? What kind of training does the doctor have? Is he or she board certified? (Board certification requires special training, as well as ongoing education.) Which hospital does the doctor work with? Are there other doctors in the practice whom you may see, as well? What is the practice's after-hours policy? How do they handle emergencies? If your family has special health concerns, be sure to ask about the doctor's experience in that area.

Taking the time to find the right primary care doctor is important. That's because, ideally, you'll be together for a long time. He or she will be your partner in making many smart health decisions. When routine illnesses occur, you know where to turn. And, if complex health issues arise, your primary care doctor can help coordinate medical care with other doctors, as needed.

31 ▶ PLAN FOR YOUR NEXT VISIT

A little planning can help you make the most of each doctor visit. Before you go, take the time to gather some key information.

Make notes about your questions and concerns in order of importance. Start with a list of symptoms. Include the dates and times they appeared. List any known triggers. Note whether the symptoms have gotten better or worse. Be sure to let your doctor know if you've taken any over-the-counter (OTC) medicines for relief. Note if the medicines worked. It's also smart to show your doctor a current list of all the prescription and OTC medications you take regularly. Don't forget to include any vitamins, supplements and herbal remedies.

Bring an up-to-date health history with you, if you have it. If you've had any recent tests, bring the results so that you can talk with your doctor about them. Note any allergies you have. See Part Three of this book, Page 207, for tools that can help you collect this kind of information.

32 ▶ MAKE THE MOST OF YOUR TIME TOGETHER

When you meet with your doctor, try to be clear and brief. Focus on the most important facts about your condition. Here are a few tips that may help:

Be clear. Try to be specific when you talk about your symptoms. For example, you may be tired all the time. And, that's the main reason for seeing your doctor. But, you also may be sleeping poorly. Perhaps you've gained or lost weight. Or, maybe you're having more headaches. It's important to tell exactly what's going on.

Be complete. It's natural to feel shy or nervous about sensitive topics. But, don't hold back. Doctors hear it all. Your doctor needs complete information in order to help you. This may include knowing your sexual history. It also may include your alcohol and drug use.

Ask questions and take notes. Ask about tests and what the results may mean. Find out about the possible side effects of a new medicine. Ask about any procedures coming up. Be sure to take notes. Or, bring along a family member or friend who can help remember details.

Prepare for follow-up. Before you leave, ask some key questions. How will you get answers to follow-up questions? When will you get your test results? Does the doctor have brochures or handouts so you can learn more about your health condition?

33 ▶ KNOW YOUR TEAM

Your primary care doctor is the main player on your health care team. But, he or she is supported by many other professionals. They play an important role in your well-being, too. These are just a few:

Nurses. These health care professionals support your doctor in a wide variety of ways. They provide care, expertise and comfort. They can answer questions about prevention, wellness and illness. And, they can tell you about other medical support services that may help. Some might even say that nurses are the unsung heroes of the health care team. Take advantage of this great resource.

Nurse practitioners (NPs). These registered nurses have additional training. NPs can diagnose and treat illnesses. They also can order and read lab tests and X-rays. They're able to prescribe medications. Some NPs work with doctors as part of the practice. Others can serve as primary providers in family medicine, pediatrics, internal medicine and geriatrics.

Physician assistants (PAs). These professionals are licensed to practice medicine with a doctor's supervision. They can diagnose and treat illnesses. PAs also can write prescriptions. They also assist in surgery.

Pharmacists. Your pharmacist is a great source of information. Not sure if you should take your medicine on an empty stomach? Forgot to ask your doctor if it's safe to take a cold remedy at the same time? Call your pharmacist. When you use one pharmacy, you get additional benefits. They'll have all of your prescriptions listed in their computer system. So, they'll let you know of any dangerous combinations. This is especially important if you are seeing more than one doctor.

34 ▸ UNDERSTAND YOUR TESTS

Medical tests are important tools. They help your doctor diagnose your condition. Tests also help him or her decide the best treatment options. Be an informed health care consumer by asking these questions:
- Why is the test being done?
- What will it involve?
- Are there any special instructions, such as fasting beforehand?
- When will the results be back?

If you don't get your test results when promised, call and ask for them. If you think your test results don't seem right, talk with your doctor about it. Don't forget, check with your health plan about coverage for tests and procedures.

35 ▸ TAKE ADVANTAGE OF A NURSE HELP LINE

When you're sick, you'll likely see your doctor. But, there are times when you may have general questions. Or, you might not be sure if a doctor visit is needed for some symptoms. That's where nurse information services, also called nurse help lines, can really help.

Some health plans and employers provide this type of resource. They're easy to use. Typically, you can call a nurse any time, 24 hours a day, to ask health questions. Some hospitals and doctor's offices also offer some version of a nurse help line. This is a great way to get more information about a health issue. The nurse can even help you make a list of questions to ask your doctor.

36 ▶ CONSIDER GETTING A SECOND OPINION

There are times when you may want to get another doctor's opinion. Some examples include:

• Your case is difficult or your condition is rare.
• Your doctor wants you to have major surgery.
• You've been told you have a life-threatening disease, such as cancer or heart disease.
• You have more than one medical problem.
• You want to better understand treatment options.
• You want to feel more confident about your health decision.

Don't be afraid to ask your doctor for a referral for a second opinion. Many people think their doctors will be unhappy or offended. In fact, most doctors view a second opinion as an important tool. It can help you make smart decisions about your health care. Remember to check with your health plan. Ask if second-opinion visits are covered.

37 ▶ PREVENT MEDICATION ERRORS

Medication errors harm at least 1.5 million Americans every year, according to the National Academies Institute of Medicine. These steps can help you stay safe:

• Make sure you understand why your doctor prescribed the drug.
• Tell your doctor and pharmacist about allergies or any reactions you've had.

- Also, tell them about all prescription and OTC medications you take. Include herbal remedies and supplements.
- Let them know about any recent changes to your condition.
- If possible, try to use the same pharmacy every time. Doing so may help prevent errors. It will also help your pharmacist spot any potentially dangerous combinations.

Most medication errors involve the wrong medication or the wrong dose. At the pharmacy, check the medicine you receive before you pay for it. Read the label. Is your name correct? Is it the medicine your doctor prescribed? Is the dose right? If something seems wrong, ask the pharmacist. If you use a mail-order prescription service, call if you have any questions. Ask to speak with a pharmacist.

38 ▶ LEARN MORE

If you have symptoms you don't recognize or understand, you may be tempted to go online and do your own research. Be sure to use the most reliable sites. And, always talk about your findings with your doctor. How do you know a site is reliable? Look for the following:

Sites sponsored by the federal government. The Web address always ends with .gov. The National Institutes of Health (nih.gov) or the Centers for Disease Control and Prevention (cdc.gov) are very reliable sites.

Sites that end in .edu. Universities or medical schools run these.

Sites that end in .org. These tend to focus on research and public education. Not-for-profit professional groups often run them. The American Cancer Society (cancer.org) or the American Diabetes Association (diabetes.org) are good examples.

5 Habits That Improve Your Health

Some habits, such as walking the dog after reading the morning newspaper, can be great for your overall health and happiness. But, other habits, such as smoking cigarettes or not getting enough sleep, may put your well-being at risk. Here are smart ways to help you lead a healthier, happier life.

39 ▶ GET A GOOD NIGHT'S SLEEP

A full night's rest doesn't just leave you feeling great in the morning. It also may better your health and your relationships. Not surprisingly, getting too little sleep may have the opposite effect. About 60 million adults have frequent insomnia, according to the National Institutes of Health. And, some 20 million people say they have sleeping problems from time to time. The results are serious.

Lack of sleep may play a role in obesity, depression and diabetes. It may even affect your relationships. The National Sleep Foundation has found that 20 percent of Americans are having less sex because they're too tired. Other studies show that people who don't get six hours of sleep a night are more likely to be obese. The same is true for those who sleep more than nine hours. To make sure you're getting the right amount of sleep, try these tips:

Make a sleep schedule. Most adults need seven or eight hours of sleep per night. The average American spends six hours and 55 minutes in bed per night. But, not all of that time is spent sleeping. A regular sleep schedule can help. Try to go to bed and wake up at roughly the same time every day. The goal is to get the same amount of shut-eye—and enough—every night. This means on weekends, too.

Create a peaceful environment. It sounds basic, but a comfortable sleeping area really is important. Most adults find that sleeping in a cool, quiet, dark room makes it easier to sleep soundly. Try turning on a fan for white noise. This can block out traffic and other sounds. And, it may help you fall asleep more quickly.

Squash sleep stealers. Caffeine, cigarettes and alcohol may hurt sleep quality. Cutting out caffeine after lunch will help your body wind down by bedtime. Quitting smoking altogether will help, too. And, don't pour yourself a nightcap. It'll rob you of sleep.

Follow a sleep routine. Start by making your bedroom a no-work zone. Don't check e-mail, watch TV or talk on the phone in the bedroom. About 30 to 60 minutes before bedtime, start unwinding. Dim the lights. Turn off your TV. Turn on some soft music. This will let your body slow down and get ready for sleep.

Don't toss and turn. If you don't fall asleep within 20 minutes, get up and do something that's soothing to you. Read, knit or try breathing exercises. You may find that writing down your worries in a notebook helps. The idea is to take your mind off *trying* to fall asleep.

40 ▶ COPE WITH SLEEP DISORDERS

An estimated 40 million Americans have chronic sleep disorders, such as obstructive sleep apnea, restless leg syndrome (RLS) or others, according to the National Institutes of Health. The following tips can help you address some physical problems that may rob you of sleep:

Visit your doctor. Be sure to bring along a list of your medications. That's because some drugs for allergies, asthma, depression, high blood pressure and thyroid diseases may interrupt sleep. Even over-the-counter (OTC) cold products and some supplements may ruin sleep. If you think your medications are getting in the way of your rest, talk with your doctor.

At the same time, tell your doctor about any physical sensations you have at bedtime. Do you feel like bugs are crawling up and down your legs? You may have RLS. Other signs include tingling sensations or the need to move your legs constantly. RLS is common in older people. But, it may develop at any age. In some people, it's tied to conditions such as anemia, pregnancy or diabetes.

Turn down loud snoring. Snoring may rob you and your partner of valuable sleep. Also, it may be a sign of obstructive sleep apnea. Other signs are daytime fatigue, insomnia, and choking or gasping for breath at night. This condition is caused by relaxed soft tissue in the back of the throat. The tissue blocks the airway and keeps air from reaching the lungs. Those who have it may stop breathing for 10 or more seconds several times an hour. Snoring or breathing difficulties during sleep also are tied to other health problems. These include high blood pressure and heart disease. If you suffer from any of these, talk with your doctor about your sleep.

41 ▶ DRINK WITH CAUTION

Many studies tie health ailments to alcohol use. It can be hard to sort it all out. This information can help you make informed decisions about drinking responsibly. But remember, if you're pregnant, you should not drink alcohol.

Know the pros and cons. Some research shows that moderate drinking may be good for you. Red wine, for example, is rich in antioxidants. They may protect against heart disease. And, some ingredients in alcohol act like a blood thinner. They may keep blood platelets from sticking together.

But, drinking too much also may play a part in a host of medical problems. These include various cancers and liver and gastrointestinal diseases, among others.

When it comes to alcohol and diabetes, studies conflict about whether moderate alcohol use can either prevent or improve Type 2 diabetes. But, we know this: If you take insulin shots or diabetes medication—whatever type of diabetes you have—alcohol may raise your risk of low blood sugar (hypoglycemia). If you have any of the medical conditions listed here, or other health issues, be sure to ask your doctor if you should drink at all.

Think moderation. That means no more than one drink a day for women and two for men. One drink equals a 12-ounce beer, an 8-ounce malt liquor beverage, a 5-ounce glass of wine or a 1.5-ounce shot of 80-proof distilled spirits or liquor.

Avoid the deadly mix. Prescription and nonprescription drugs mixed with alcohol can be deadly. Even mixing herbal medications with alcohol carries health risks. So, don't drink while taking any kind of medication. Harmful effects of mixing may include vomiting, fainting, internal bleeding, and breathing and heart problems.

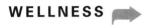

Notice signs. If you or a loved one drinks regularly to relax, fall asleep or avoid dealing with pain, it may be a sign of a drinking problem. Talk with your doctor for advice.

A Time to Say No to Alcohol

You know drinking and driving don't mix. Taking OTC meds with alcohol also has serious health consequences.

When combined with alcohol:

- Nonsteroidal anti-inflammatory drugs (NSAIDs) and other pain relievers may cause ulcers, stomach bleeding and liver problems.
- Acetaminophen may increase your risk of liver damage.
- Allergy, cold and flu medications may result in drowsiness and dizziness. They also pose a greater risk of overdose.
- Heartburn and sour stomach remedies may increase heart rate and cause sudden changes in blood pressure.

---

42 STOP SMOKING

Cigarette smoking causes nearly 90 percent of all lung-cancer deaths and 30 percent of all cancer deaths, according to the American Cancer Society. Lung cancer is one of the most difficult to treat. Mouth, throat and bladder cancer also are tied to smoking.

But, smoking's bad impact on your health isn't limited to cancer. It's also linked to bronchitis, emphysema, heart disease, aneurysms and stroke, to name a few. If you're pregnant, don't smoke—and avoid secondhand smoke.

The good news is that the moment you quit smoking, your health risks are lowered, according to the American Lung Association (ALA). While it takes three days for nicotine to leave your body, your health will improve immediately. Take a look at these short- and long-term benefits of quitting, according to the ALA:

Within 20 minutes of your last cigarette: Nicotine starts to leave your body. Your blood pressure will drop.

After eight hours: Carbon monoxide and oxygen in your blood reach normal levels.

After 24 hours: The risk of a heart attack goes down.

After 48 hours: Your senses of taste and smell get better.

Two weeks to three months after quitting: Your circulation gets better. Your lungs work better, too.

Within the first nine months: Coughing, sinus congestion, tiredness and shortness of breath all go down.

Five to 15 years after quitting: Your risk of stroke is brought down to the same level as that of a lifelong nonsmoker.

After 15 years: Your risk of getting coronary heart disease is lowered to the same level as that of a lifelong nonsmoker. Your risk of dying is now nearly the same as that of a nonsmoker.

If threats to your health aren't reason enough, think about the other costs: Cigarettes are expensive. Also, smoking causes wrinkles. More important, consider the impact on loved ones exposed to your secondhand smoke. In nonsmokers, secondhand smoke can trigger an asthma attack. It can lead to lung and heart damage. It can even lead to lung cancer in nonsmokers. In fact, the U.S. Environmental Protection Agency classifies secondhand smoke as a human carcinogen. That's why, more and more, laws ban smoking in public places.

Preparing to Quit

Here are proven tips from Smokefree.gov that may make it easier for you to join the growing ranks of former cigarette smokers:

Before You Quit:
- Learn from the past. If you've tried to quit in the past and failed, take steps to avoid similar problems this time.
- Talk with your doctor about nicotine-replacement methods. Learn how to use them. Research all your options.
- Write down why you want to quit. Keep it in a visible spot.
- Ask family and friends for their support.
- Stock up on healthful snacks to reach for when temptation hits.

Day One:
- Throw away all cigarettes, lighters and ashtrays.
- Practice deep breathing. When the urge to smoke hits, breathe deeply and exhale slowly.
- Spend time with nonsmoking friends. And, start a new hobby.
- When the urge to light up strikes, talk to an understanding friend. Find someone who will encourage you to succeed.

The First Few Days:
- Spend time with nonsmokers. Tell your smoker friends you're quitting and need their support.
- Make your home a smoke-free zone—and post signs.
- Avoid going to places where smoking is allowed.
- Avoid alcohol. It decreases your willpower and increases the odds of your lighting up.

The First Month:
- Reward yourself by putting aside the money you've saved by not buying cigarettes. Spend it on something fun and special.
- Learn to say, "No." If someone offers you a cigarette, say, "No, thanks." If you're tempted to buy a pack and smoke just one, don't do it. Remind yourself of how far you've come.

43 ► AVOID DRUG ABUSE

People don't plan to become drug addicts. Drug abuse usually begins with sampling. That's when people try a drug once to see what it's like. Certain drugs—both legal and illegal—may make you feel good for a moment. But, repeated use will affect how your brain works.

After addiction has set in, the brain will demand the addictive ingredient again and again. Research proves that long-term drug use changes your brain's ability to function normally. These changes last long after a person stops using drugs. It's worth pointing out that addiction is not a character flaw or weakness.

Some pain medications may be particularly addictive. If your pain medicine has stopped working, talk with your doctor. Don't increase the dosage on your own. If you suspect that you or a loved one is becoming dependent on a drug, talk with your doctor about other options. If you need to break an addiction to drugs, get professional help. You can contact an employee assistance program or attend Narcotics Anonymous meetings. A good source of information is the Substance Abuse Treatment Facility Locator. It's a searchable directory of more than 11,000 national treatment programs. Visit www.findtreatment.samhsa.gov.

Drug Misuse and Prescription Medicines

Drug abuse involves more than just street drugs. It often involves prescription and OTC medications. An estimated 20 percent of Americans have used prescription drugs for nonmedical purposes, according to the National Institute on Drug Abuse.

Many people don't realize they're misusing their medications. Patients ages 65 and older often take too much of their medicine by accident. This may cause dangerous drug interactions or overdoses. Some people may take more pills than prescribed to deal with pain. Others may be using medications that were prescribed for someone else.

8 Safe Tips for Home & Away

From food poisoning to road rage, safety challenges are part of everyday life. But, you can lower your risk by planning ahead and making safe choices. This chapter shines a light on simple strategies for addressing common safety hazards.

44 ▶ PROTECT YOURSELF FROM FIRE

If a fire breaks out in your home, there's more to fear than flames. Smoke and toxic gases may spread farther and faster than fire or heat. Inhaling either one could be deadly. Here are key ways to prevent—and escape from—home fires:

Install and maintain smoke detectors. Working smoke detectors are a must in every home. Some alarms respond best to smoldering fires. Others react more to flaming fires. Ideally, you should look for one that alerts you to both. These are known as dual-sensor alarms. Whatever type you buy, look for a model that meets the Underwriters Laboratories Inc. (UL) standard. It will say so on the packaging. Be sure to follow the directions for testing and replacing the battery. Doing so every six months is a good rule of thumb.

Have an escape plan. Working smoke alarms alert you to fire threats. They give you time to get out quickly and safely. But, having an escape plan is also necessary. In fact, experts advise having *two* escape routes for every room. This is in case the first way out is blocked. If you're in a room above ground level, you may need to use a fire escape. If that's not an option, you may want to think about buying a UL-classified portable escape ladder. These ladders fit over your home's windowsills. Read the instructions. And, practice using the ladder.

Safety experts recommend that families practice their escape plans ahead of time—and often. An important part of the plan is to choose a safe spot where everyone will meet once you're all out of harm's way. This is to make sure that each family member is accounted for.

Reduce fire risks. Fire can start anywhere in your home. Here are some smart things you can do to reduce the risk:

Cooking. This is the most common cause of home fires. When cooking, keep a close eye on the stove and oven. Roll up your sleeves and keep clothing away from the burners. Store spoons, spatulas and spoon rests off to the side. The goal is to avoid having to reach directly over a hot stove. If children are in the house, try to cook on the back burners. And, turn pot handles toward the back of the stove. Or, put in a safety guard to stop wandering fingers from reaching the stove top. Better yet, set up a kid-free zone while cooking. And, enforce it.

Heating or cooling equipment. The second most common cause is heating, ventilation or air-conditioning (HVAC) equipment that isn't working right. So, be sure licensed professionals check your home's HVAC units every year. If your home has a fireplace, have the chimney and flue cleaned at least once a year. And, only use portable heaters that meet the safety standards of a national testing agency such as the UL. Be sure to turn off all space heaters before going to bed or when you leave the room.

Appliances and fixtures. Every so often, go through the house and do a safety check. Don't leave on appliances that might pose a safety threat. Irons and coffee makers are good examples. Look at electrical cords and lights to see if any stiff, frayed or cracked wires need to be replaced. Make sure all your light bulbs have wattages no higher than what's recommended on the fixture. Otherwise, they may overheat. Keep paper and fabric away from light bulbs and fixtures. Don't overload extension cords. Too many appliances plugged into one cord can be dangerous. Instead, consider having a licensed electrician put in new outlets where you need them most.

Candles and cigarettes. These also present fire hazards. Keep lit candles, matches and lighters away from children. Never leave candles burning when no one's in the room. Keep them away from paper, fabric and other flammable materials. During power outages, use flashlights instead of candles. If you smoke, always use an ashtray. And, never smoke in bed. Better yet, quit smoking—for your health and your safety!

Better than Batteries

Battery-powered smoke alarms are the simplest to install. But, if you're having a new home built or renovating your current home, you may want a smoke alarm system that's hooked up to your home's wiring system. The best hard-wired systems include battery backup in case of power failures. This means you'll still have to check and change your smoke alarm batteries regularly.

45 ▶ PREVENT CARBON MONOXIDE POISONING

Odorless and colorless, carbon monoxide (CO) gas is a more common threat than you might imagine. It's given off by fuel-burning appliances. These include gas stoves, water heaters, furnaces, boilers and kerosene heaters. Fireplaces and wood stoves also release the gas. CO may leak from a faulty furnace or heater. A blocked chimney or flue is another source. More than 500 Americans die each year from accidentally inhaling this poisonous gas. Many more develop flu-like symptoms that are never attributed to CO.

To lower the threat of CO poisoning, know the symptoms. Fatigue, nausea, dizziness, confusion and shortness of breath may be early signs of dangerous CO levels. Severe signs of CO exposure include vomiting, irregular heartbeat, breathing difficulties and loss of consciousness. If you or anyone in your home has any possible symptoms of CO poisoning, move everyone outside for fresh air right away. Then, call 911.

To lower the risk of CO exposure in your home, put in CO detectors. Place at least one on each level. Be sure one is near every bedroom. Choose models that meet UL Standard 2034. If the alarm sounds, don't ignore it. Push the alarm's reset button. Then, move outside. If anyone is showing signs of CO poisoning, call 911. Quick medical attention is key. If everyone feels fine, open windows and doors. Turn off all fuel-burning appliances and heaters. Before returning to your home, have a qualified technician check your appliances and chimneys.

Make sure your appliances are in good repair. Gas, oil, kerosene, wood and charcoal appliances that are properly installed, maintained and inspected will release very small, harmless amounts of CO. But, those emissions may build to dangerous levels if the appliance isn't working right. As stated earlier, have your furnace serviced every year. And, if you think something is wrong with your stove or water heater, call a professional. Also, try to have appliances with vents, such as dryers, direct fumes outside.

Use other appliances with safety in mind, too. Never use a charcoal grill indoors, for example. Don't use a gas range or oven to heat your home. If you decide to use an unvented kerosene or propane space heater, use it only while someone is awake and in the room.

Don't let cars or trucks idle when not in use. Never leave a motor running in a garage. This is true even if the garage door is open. And, don't use gas-powered lawn tools, small engines or generators in a closed space.

46 ▶ AVOID FOOD POISONING

Stomachaches, diarrhea, vomiting and fever are signs of food poisoning. Often, these symptoms go away fairly quickly. But, they may become severe. At times, they even may require emergency care. The Centers for Disease Control and Prevention encourages people who think they may have a food-related illness to call the health department. Doing so may help prevent others from getting it. Here are a few easy ways to lower the risk of most cases of food poisoning:

Be smart about packaged foods. Check expiration or sell-by dates. This will help you avoid accidentally preparing or eating out-of-date items.

Wash all fresh fruits and vegetables. Scrub firm produce, such as melons and cucumbers, under running water. Use a clean produce brush. Rinse delicate fruits, such as berries. Dry fruits and vegetables with a clean paper towel. This will help reduce the amount of bacteria.

Safely handle meat. When grocery shopping, keep meats, poultry and seafood separate from other foods. This means both in your cart and in your bags. Keep meats chilled until cooking. If you plan to use them soon, store meats and poultry in containers or sealed plastic bags in the refrigerator. Freeze ground meats, poultry or seafood within two days of purchase. Freeze other refrigerated meats within four or five days of purchase. Never let meat marinate at room temperature, only while refrigerated. Before cooking, fully defrost frozen meats, poultry and seafood in the microwave or refrigerator. Rinsing under cold running water also works. Don't thaw food on the counter.

Guard against cross contamination. Keep raw meats, poultry, seafood and their juices away from ready-to-eat and precooked foods. Never place cooked foods back on a plate or cutting board that previously held raw foods. Don't reuse utensils, cutting boards or other kitchen equipment that's been exposed to raw meats or other foods. Wash them well with soap and hot water first.

Pay attention to temperatures. When making a meal, keep hot foods at 140° F or higher. Reheat cooked foods to at least 165° F. Bring sauces, soups and gravies to a boil when reheating. Keep cold foods at 40° F or lower. Don't miss the picnic and party tips below.

Keep kitchen tools safe. Sanitize cutting boards with bleach diluted in water. Mix 1 teaspoon of bleach with 1 quart of hot water. Wash dish towels weekly using hot water. Be sure your refrigerator is set at 40° F or lower. Set your freezer temperature at 0° F.

Be smart when storing leftovers. Throw out any perishable food that's been left at room temperature for longer than two hours. Also, throw out food that's been sitting out for one hour at a temperature higher than 90° F. Divide large amounts of leftovers into small, shallow containers. This will help the food cool quickly in the refrigerator. Remove the stuffing from poultry and other meats right away. Refrigerate it in its own container.

Tips for Picnics and Parties

Don't forget the hot-and-cold rules when laying out food for your next gathering. Keep foods hot by using chafing dishes, steam tables, warming trays or slow cookers. Set cold dishes on ice. Or, put them in a cooler:

- Use enough ice or ice packs to keep the food at 40° F or lower.
- Keep the cooler out of the sun.
- Try to keep the lid shut as much as possible.
- Put meat and drinks in separate coolers. People reach for drinks often. The meat needs to stay as cool as possible.

Safe Cooking Temperatures

This chart and a food thermometer will help keep you safe.

FOOD	FINISHED COOKING
Eggs	Cook until yolk and white are firm
Egg casseroles, custards and sauces	160° F

Poultry

Ground chicken and turkey	165° F
Whole chicken and turkey	180° F
Dark-meat chicken and turkey	180° F
Breast-meat chicken and turkey	170° F
Duck and goose	180° F
Poultry stuffing	165° F (whether cooked alone or in a bird)

Beef, Lamb and Veal

Ground beef, lamb and veal	160° F
Fresh beef, lamb and veal • Medium-rare • Medium • Well-done	 145° F 160° F 170° F

Pork

Ground pork	160° F
Fresh pork • Medium • Well-done	 160° F 170° F

Ham

Fresh (raw)	160° F
Fully cooked	Reheat to 140° F

Seafood

Fish	Cook until opaque and flakes easily
Crab, lobster, shrimp	Cook until shell reddens and flesh is pearly
Clams, mussels, oysters	Cook until shells open

Leftovers

All leftovers	Reheat to 165° F

Source: Adapted from the USDA Food Safety and Inspection Service

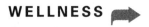

47 GIVE GERMS THE BOOT

Keep surfaces clean to help stop the spread of germs that cause colds, the flu and other infections. This is true for your home, work area and car. Try these tips:

Choose a germ-fighting cleaner. Harmful bacteria may be found on kitchen countertops, tables and bathroom surfaces. A few of the bad ones are E. coli, salmonella, staphylococcus and streptococcus. Your phone, doorknobs and remote controls also are germ sources. Cleaning removes dirt and debris. But, only sanitizing kills germs. Store-bought germ-killing products will work. Or, make your own sanitizer. Mix 1 teaspoon of bleach with 1 quart of hot water.

Use a clean sponge, cloth or paper towel. Sponges are a breeding ground for bacteria. To keep yours clean, run them through the dishwasher with the dry cycle left on. Another option is to microwave your damp sponge once a day for 60 seconds. Or, skip the sponge and clean with paper towels and a disinfectant spray.

Wash your hands frequently. Wash under warm water for 20 seconds—the amount of time it takes to hum "Happy Birthday" twice. Any soap will do. Washing rubs and rinses viruses and bacteria off your skin.

Carry antibacterial wipes. These are great to have handy when running errands. Use them to wipe down cart handles. Or, use them on your hands after pumping gas. And, at your workplace, they're great for cleaning your phone, keyboard and desktop.

The Best Way to Kill Germs

Gently, but vigorously, wash your hands with soap and warm water for 20 seconds before handling food. Remember to wash your hands again after handling raw meats, poultry, fish or eggs. And, always wash your hands before eating.

---

48 TAKE SAFETY PERSONALLY

We all want to feel safe and secure as we go through our day. These simple steps may help:

Consider a self-defense course. Everyone worries about becoming a victim of crime. But, don't just worry—take action. Enroll in a self-defense course. It can really boost your confidence. You can learn how to get away, and more. Remember, the most important thing you can do is try to keep from fighting an attacker. Give a mugger your wallet, for example. Many times, trusting your gut is your best defense.

Keep your home secure. Install good locks on windows and outside doors. Don't forget to lock them! Put in a peephole that lets you see a large area in front of your door. Use lights to brighten entryways, pathways, stairwells and parking areas. Consider adding lights that switch on automatically at dusk or when you come home.

Don't open the door to a stranger. Ask all repairmen for photo identification. They can slip an ID card under the door or hold it up to a window. If you didn't request a visit or service, call the phone number on the ID card. Ask who the person is and why he's at your house.

Take care when walking alone. Whenever practical, try to walk with someone. The safest routes tend to be busy, well-lit streets. If you do find yourself walking alone, stay alert to your surroundings. Try to look busy and confident. Take particular care when using a shortcut or on secluded paths. At these times, don't talk on your cell phone or use headphones.

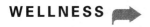
Park in well-lit areas at night. If you're parking during daylight but will return to your car when it's dark, look around to be sure there are lights nearby. At work, park near coworkers, if possible. Then, you can walk to your cars together at the end of the day.

Car trouble? Pull off the road and stay in your car. If you have a cell phone, call for help. Put a white cloth or bag on your antenna or handle. Passing motorists will see this as a distress signal. If someone stops to help, stay in your car and ask her to call the police. Or, let her know that help is already on the way.

Create a Lifeline with ICE

Did you know you can turn your cell phone into an emergency-contact device? Program it with an In Case of Emergency (ICE) name and contact number. Store it under the acronym ICE. Emergency personnel know to look for this cue. In an emergency, an ICE number may be a lifeline.

---

49 ▶ MAKE A FIRST-AID KIT

Everyone should have a well-organized first-aid kit. The best kit is easy to carry and easy to find things in. A toolbox is a good choice. Make one for both your home and car. Use the following guidelines:

Include three lists. Make a list of emergency telephone numbers. Use the form found on Page 208. Include your doctor and the Poison Help hotline (1-800-222-1222). Make a second list of the medications your family takes. There's a handy form on Page 214. Don't forget to note any allergies. Finally, keep a checklist of the kit's contents for easy updating.

Stock it well. Include basics such as bandages and instant-activating cold packs. For a more complete list, see Your First-Aid Kit: The Essentials, Page 209.

Update it yearly. Review and revise your lists as needed. Check expiration dates on all medications and replace as needed.

50 ▶ BE A SAFE DRIVER

There are many dangers on the road. These basics may help you keep safe:

Don't be distracted. When you're driving, don't do anything else. This includes eating and drinking. Avoid talking a lot with other people in the car. Don't read or text message when you're driving. If you must use your cell phone, pull off the road. Getting too absorbed by the radio, music or a DVD are other dangerous distractions.

Buckle up. One in five people admits to driving without wearing a seat belt. Nearly 6,000 Americans are killed each year because they weren't wearing seat belts. And, 80,000 more are seriously hurt. These grim statistics are from a 2005 National Mason-Dixon poll conducted for Drive for Life, the National Safe Driving Test and Initiative. So, buckle up every time you get into the car, no matter how short the trip.

Don't drive when you're sleepy. About 71,000 people each year are hurt in accidents caused by someone falling asleep at the wheel, according to the National Highway Traffic Safety Administration. You're at a higher risk if you slept less than six hours the night before or if you've been awake for 20 hours or longer. People who work more than one job, work the night shift, or often drive between midnight and 6 a.m. are also at a higher risk. On long trips, take a break every two hours.

Focusing on the Road?

Nearly 98 percent of people say they're safe drivers. But, 72 percent admit to multitasking while driving. Eighty-one percent talk on their cell phones and 18 percent text message while driving. Source: Nationwide Insurance

---

Don't drive when angry or upset. You'll be less likely to pay attention to the road. If an angry driver confronts you—with mean gestures or aggressive driving—ignore him or her. Safely get out of the way.

Keep your distance. Maintain enough space between you and the car ahead of you. This will allow for emergency stopping or maneuvering. This distance will depend on your speed, the weather and road conditions.

Be aware of what's around you. Be on the lookout for people and other cars. Pay close attention at intersections. Check your blind spots. And, always use your turn signals.

Take steps to make your trip safer and calmer. Planning ahead can help you avoid heavy traffic, bad weather and roads where drivers tend to speed. If you belong to an emergency road service, bring your member card with you.

Stick to the speed limit. Going faster or slower than the speed limit on major highways is unsafe.

Avoid tire trouble. A car with underinflated or worn tires won't perform well when stopping, turning or handling in bad weather. You can't tell by looking if your tires have lost pressure. So, be sure to check them often. You can do this with your own tire gauge or at a gas station. Inflate your tires to the pressure recommended by the manufacturer. You will usually find this information inside the driver's-side door frame or door post. It's also wise to check your tire treads for wear and tear. Rotate your tires according to the owner's manual.

Keep on rolling. Keep your gas tank filled, but don't stop there. You'll drive more safely and comfortably if your car is tuned-up regularly, too. Be sure to follow your car manufacturer's recommended maintenance schedule. This will help you avoid car troubles down the road. You'll find the schedule in your owner's manual.

Get a clear view of the road. If you need distance glasses or contacts, always wear them when driving. Be sure your prescription is up to date. Keep your windshield and your back and side windows clean on the inside and outside. Clean your car's mirrors and headlights, too. Be sure your headlights are working. And, ask your mechanic to see if they're aimed correctly. Sit high enough in your seat to see at least 10 feet of road in front of your vehicle.

Replace used air bags. If your air bag is released in an accident, be sure to have it replaced. An air bag can't be reused. It should be replaced with a new one that's right for the make and model of your car.

Keeping an Edge

Drivers ages 65 to 74 are less likely to have crashes than younger drivers. This may be because they're less likely to drive drunk or in unsafe conditions. But, the risk of accidents and fatalities rises after age 74. This is due to age-related vision changes. Another reason is that older people often drive cars that are older and less safe. To keep your driving edge, consider taking a driver-safety refresher course. This will help make you a safer driver. And, it may lower your auto insurance rates. Source: Centers for Disease Control and Prevention and AARP

---

51 ▶ TRAVEL SAFELY

Whether you're traveling to a nearby city or around the world, personal safety should be a top priority whenever you're away from home. The Centers for Disease Control and Prevention's Web site has lots of useful advice in this area. Vaccines and preventive medicines may be needed for certain countries. Visit www.cdc.gov/travel for more information. Here are additional travel safety tips:

Let your doctor know your plans. Tell him or her where you're going and when you're leaving. He or she can advise you about any vaccinations or preventive medicines you may need. Your doctor also can tell you about other smart measures to take. Depending on where you're going, this might include things such as packing insect repellent or water purification tablets.

Check your health plan. Find out if it covers medical care abroad. If you're in a remote area or country where health care facilities aren't up to par, does your plan cover medical evacuation? You may want to buy short-term health insurance that specifically covers emergency services abroad.

Carry your medications. Pack them in your carry-on bag. Bring enough for your entire trip, plus a few days' extra. Keep medicines in their original labeled containers. This will help you avoid problems when passing through customs and airport security. Bring copies of your prescriptions. If you take an unusual medication or a narcotic, bring a letter from your doctor that states your need for this drug. Wear a bracelet or necklace describing any special medical conditions. Also, carry that information in your wallet.

Alert friends and family. Give family members, friends and important contacts a detailed trip itinerary. Let them know how to reach you. Make two copies of your passport identification page, airline tickets, driver's license and the credit cards you're bringing. Leave one copy with family or friends at home. Pack the other in your luggage.

Get up to speed. When traveling abroad, find out about travel warnings and alerts by logging onto the U.S. Department of State's travel Web site. Go to www.travel.state.gov.

Stay cool, comfortable and well-hydrated. Drink enough water to stay hydrated. Avoid too much alcohol and caffeine. Wear a hat and sunglasses to shield yourself from the sun's rays. And, comfortable shoes are a must for sightseeing. During intense heat, try to stay in air-conditioned spaces as much as possible.

Avoiding Getting Sick on Vacation

Many visitors to foreign locales bring home an unwanted souvenir: traveler's diarrhea. You can cut your chances by remembering the four P's when it comes to food: make sure it's peelable, packaged, purified or piping hot.

---

PART TWO

34 SYMPTOM SOLUTIONS

How to Make Smart Health Care Choices

MAKING HEALTH CARE DECISIONS MEANS MORE THAN choosing a doctor or health plan. It means making smart choices every day. This is especially true when illnesses or injuries occur. But, knowing what choice to make for yourself or your family isn't always easy. For instance, emergency care might seem like a good way to get fast treatment. However, in some situations, you may spend many hours in the waiting room and then pay high out-of-pocket fees. And, it's not uncommon to wonder whether you really need to see a doctor or if you can treat a health concern at home. This symptoms section can help take the guesswork out of making health choices. Keep in mind that you should never try to diagnose yourself. And, these tips should not replace your doctor's advice. Instead, use them as an important tool that can help put the power of choice in your hands.

ABDOMINAL PAIN

UNDERSTANDING YOUR SYMPTOMS

Abdominal pain may come from something as simple as eating a heavy or spicy meal. But, it also may be a sign of a more serious condition. The following are examples of some of the more common reasons for your pain. Be aware that sometimes people may show different symptoms from the classic ones described below. Also, this list doesn't include all causes of abdominal pain.

- Appendicitis is most often felt as a dull-then-sharp pain that moves from the navel to the lower-right abdomen.
- Diverticulitis is the result of an infection in pouches of the large intestine wall. Sufferers may have fever, pain, tenderness and constipation.
- Gallstones may cause pain in the right upper abdomen. The pain may radiate to your back. Sufferers also may have vomiting, heartburn or indigestion.
- Gastroenteritis is an inflammation of the stomach and intestine. Vomiting, diarrhea and cramping are the common signs.
- Heartburn is felt as a burning sensation in your chest or throat. Frequent sufferers actually may have gastroesophageal reflux disease, or GERD.
- Irritable bowel syndrome (IBS) is a chronic disorder. It includes bouts of cramping, bloating and possibly constipation alternating with diarrhea.
- Ovarian cysts are usually benign ovarian tumors. They may cause pain if they rupture, bleed, twist or push on nearby organs. A constant dull ache in your pelvis is common.
- Pancreatitis—or an inflamed pancreas—is marked by severe pain in your upper abdomen that may radiate to

your back. Fever, nausea or vomiting also may be present.

• Pelvic infections—including pelvic inflammatory disease (PID) and endometritis—are most commonly felt as pain and tenderness. Fever and sometimes an abnormal vaginal discharge also may be present.

• Peptic ulcers result from a sore that develops in the stomach lining. It causes burning stomach pain that may come and go. It may hurt more on an empty stomach.

• Peritonitis is an inflammation of the lining of the abdomen. It's usually caused by a ruptured organ, such as the appendix. Pain is often coupled with fever and nausea. And, the pain may increase with movement.

Because abdominal pain is associated with a number of illnesses, including heart disease, it will most likely require a medical evaluation. This is especially true for pregnant women, adults ages 65 and older and those with a weakened immune system. See also Chest Pain, Page 110.

---

52 ▶ DECIDING YOUR NEXT STEP

CALL 911:

• You have signs of shock. This may include a rapid heartbeat, rapid breathing, low blood pressure, faintness, confusion, lack of alertness, sweating, pale skin and a weak pulse.

• You're lightheaded or faint.

• You have blood in your vomit—which may look like coffee grounds—or blood in your stool, which may appear maroon or tarry black.

SEEK EMERGENCY HELP:

• You're vomiting repeatedly with no relief from your pain.

• You have intense shaking chills—more than just shivering.

• Your abdomen feels hard, rigid and sensitive.

• Your pain gets worse when you walk or move.

• Your pain is severe or you're extremely ill.

(Continued)

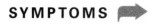

DECIDING YOUR NEXT STEP *(Continued)*

SEE YOUR DOCTOR TODAY:

- You have abdominal pain or bloating that lasts longer than two hours.
- You have a fever of more than 100.4° F.
- You have blood-streaked vomit or stools with a few streaks or specks of blood.
- You have diabetes or a weakened immune system.

CALL YOUR DOCTOR OR NURSE HELP LINE:

- Your pain has been off and on for at least two days.
- You urinate frequently or it burns when you urinate.
- You're pregnant or suspect you're pregnant.
- You have a history of abdominal surgery or a medical condition such as ulcerative colitis or bowel obstructions or adhesions.
- You experience unexplained weight loss.

TRY SELF-CARE:

- Your pain is mild and isn't accompanied by any of the symptoms above. However, if your pain persists or changes, call your doctor.

SMART ACTIONS TODAY

If your symptoms indicate emergency care:

Don't eat or drink anything. This is in case you need emergency surgery.

If your symptoms indicate self-care:

Rehydrate. If you've been vomiting, sip clear fluids frequently but slowly to prevent dehydration. Wait six hours before eating. Then, eat only small amounts of bland foods.

Ease the burn. For indigestion or heartburn, consider an antacid. Or, with your doctor's OK, take an over-the-counter histamine-2 blocker or proton pump inhibitor. If these don't help, call your doctor.

SMART ACTIONS TOMORROW

To prevent stomach ills, try the following:

Eat small, frequent meals. Large meals may trigger indigestion. So, try smaller meals five or six times a day. Also, avoid alcohol. It may erode the stomach's lining.

Fill up with fiber. A high-fiber diet helps regulate your bowels. Aim for 25 to 30 grams daily. Switch to whole-grain bread. Eat more fresh produce, legumes, beans and nuts. A fiber supplement also may help. And, try to drink water throughout the day to prevent constipation.

Keep a food diary. If you suffer from a digestive issue, track what you eat and how you feel afterward. This may help you pinpoint trigger foods. Do this for a month.

Eat yogurt. Yogurt is a wonder food for digestion. The good bacteria in yogurt, called probiotics, speed digestion. Look for *Lactobacillus bulgaricus* and *L. acidophilus,* or *contains live active cultures,* on the label.

Quick Tip

Abdominal discomfort associated with irritable bowel syndrome or heartburn may come and go. But, be alert to pain that comes on suddenly, increases or intensifies. Also, be aware of pain that feels different than usual. If this happens, call your doctor right away.

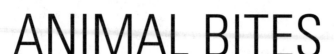

ANIMAL BITES

UNDERSTANDING YOUR SYMPTOMS

Dog bites make up most of all animal bites each year. However, cat bites are more likely to cause infections. Injuries from wild animals pose the added risk of rabies. Raccoons, bats, skunks and foxes are the most common wild animals to bite people. Don't try to catch the animal that's bitten you. Call an animal control office, the game warden or the police for help right away.

Human bites may be even more dangerous than animal bites. That's because the bacteria in the human mouth are more likely to cause infection. Plus, there's a low—but still real—risk of infection from hepatitis B, hepatitis C or HIV. So, it's important to get immediate medical attention.

---

53 ▶ DECIDING YOUR NEXT STEP

CALL 911:

- You're bleeding uncontrollably.
- You have signs of shock. This may include a rapid heartbeat, rapid breathing, low blood pressure, faintness, confusion, lack of alertness, sweating, pale skin and a weak pulse.
- You've been bitten on your head, neck, abdomen, chest or back, and the bite is deep or crushing.

SEEK EMERGENCY HELP:

- You've been bitten by a wild animal or bat.
- Your bite is deep or gaping and may require stitches.
- You have more than one bite.
- You can't feel or move the body part that's been bitten.
- The bite area is extremely swollen or bruised.

SEE YOUR DOCTOR TODAY:

- You've been bitten on your hands, feet, or near your genital area or a joint.
- Your bite came from an unfamiliar pet or a pet with an out-of-date rabies vaccination.
- The wound is swollen, hot or oozing.
- You've been bitten by a cat and develop a headache, fever, fatigue or a small bump at the bite site.
- You haven't had a tetanus shot within the past five years, you haven't completed the tetanus series, or you're not sure when you had your last tetanus shot.
- You've been exposed to—but not necessarily bitten by—a bat or rabid animal.
- You've been in close contact with any animal that was bitten by a rabid animal. Or, with any animal that had close exposure to a rabid animal.
- The site becomes numb or tingles.
- You have a weakened immune system, a chronic medical condition or vascular disease, a prosthetic valve or joint, are older than age 65, or are physically weak.
- The animal that's bitten you is behaving strangely.

CALL YOUR DOCTOR OR NURSE HELP LINE:

- You've been bitten by any animal.
- You have a cat scratch on your hand.
- Your wound hasn't healed within 10 days.

TRY SELF-CARE:

- The bite doesn't break the skin.

What to Do if Bitten

Immediately wash the wound thoroughly with soap and water. This is an important step to help prevent infection.

SMART ACTIONS TODAY

If your bite doesn't require emergency care:

Stop the bleeding. Apply pressure with a clean, dry cloth. Elevate the bite area above the heart.

Clean and bandage. Gently, but thoroughly, wash the area around the wound. Use mild soap and warm water. Then, loosely bandage. Bite wounds usually heal within 10 days.

Notify authorities. Let your local public health office know that you've been bitten.

SMART ACTIONS TOMORROW

Try these steps to discourage pets from biting, and to avoid bites:

Keep your pets healthy. Sick pets are often more aggressive than usual. Take pets to the vet if they are sick. Make sure yours are vaccinated and spayed or neutered.

Do not disturb. If your pet is eating, sleeping or caring for its young, stay away. Avoid any unfamiliar animal.

Don't move. Remain still or move very slowly if a strange dog approaches you. Avoid direct eye contact. Most times it will sniff you and then leave. If you're knocked over, curl up into a tight ball and keep still.

Cover garbage. And, don't leave pet food outside. The smell may attract stray animals.

ANXIETY

UNDERSTANDING YOUR SYMPTOMS

Many people will have a case of the jitters before a big event. But, for some people, anxiety is long-lasting and uncomfortable. And, it may take many distinct forms:

- Generalized anxiety disorder (GAD) is a state of constant worry or tension. It lasts at least six months.
- Panic disorder is marked by sudden, uncontrollable attacks of terror. These attacks involve a sense of fear and unreality. Heart pounding, shortness of breath and dizziness may go along with the attacks.
- Post-traumatic stress disorder (PTSD) results from a severely traumatic event. Soldiers and crime victims have an increased risk of having PTSD. Nightmares, flashbacks and unprovoked anger are symptoms.
- Obsessive-compulsive disorder (OCD) is marked by repeated and unwanted thoughts, or obsessions. They're often coupled with repetitious acts, or compulsions. These actions are performed to control the obsessions.
- Social anxiety disorder (SAD) is the fear of being publicly embarrassed. Sufferers try hard to avoid social settings.

Untreated, an anxiety disorder may get worse. Physically, it may lead to an increase in blood pressure. Rapid heart rate and breathing, muscle tension, nausea or diarrhea are other potential side effects. But, symptoms you think are due to anxiety actually may be due to other health problems. It's key to see your doctor for a diagnosis.

Trend Line

Anxiety disorders affect an estimated 40 million Americans, or about 18 percent of the population, each year.

Source: National Institute of Mental Health

54 ► DECIDING YOUR NEXT STEP

CALL 911:
• You're thinking about committing suicide.
• You're planning to harm someone.
• You're extremely confused or agitated.

SEE YOUR DOCTOR TODAY:
• You feel out of control.

CALL YOUR DOCTOR OR NURSE HELP LINE:
• You've been worrying excessively for several months without reason.
• Your anxiety is interfering with your daily life.

TRY SELF-CARE:
• You experience mild, short-term anxiety.

SMART ACTIONS TODAY

If your symptoms indicate self-care:

Spend time with loved ones. Surround yourself with people you enjoy. It's a great way to distract yourself.

Use relaxation techniques. Try some light exercise. Go for a walk or a swim. Regular exercise can be very helpful in coping with anxiety. Check with your doctor before starting any new exercise program. Some people find that meditation, yoga or prayer may help, too.

Try a thought-stopping technique. Once a day, set aside 10 minutes to think about nothing else but what troubles you. At the end of those 10 minutes, put away those thoughts until the next day. Over time, you may start to feel less anxious. That's because you may not be as focused on what's been bothering you.

ANXIETY ISN'T A REAL MEDICAL CONDITION
MYTH. Anxiety disorders are very real — and serious — conditions. They may develop as a result of your genetic makeup, an imbalance of chemical messengers in your brain, a distressing environment or upsetting event.

SMART ACTIONS TOMORROW

Tips to help prevent normal feelings of anxiety from escalating:

Find a support group. These groups provide a safe place to express your feelings. You'll be with others who also are experiencing anxiety.

Talk it out. Express your feelings with someone you trust and can talk with openly.

Avoid crutches. Anxiety often leads to unhealthful coping mechanisms. Smoking and overeating are two examples. Excessive caffeine use and abusing alcohol and drugs are others. Such crutches may cause *more* anxiety.

Seek help. If your anxiety persists, make an appointment with a mental health professional. Ask your primary care doctor for a recommendation. Or, contact a mental health association or community mental health center.

BACK PAIN— LOW

UNDERSTANDING YOUR SYMPTOMS

Low back pain is second only to colds and flu as the most common cause of doctor visits. In fact, about 15 percent of Americans are coping with low back pain at any given moment. The good news is that 50 percent of back pain episodes almost completely resolve within two weeks. And, 80 percent of them get better within six weeks.

Pain in the lower back is a symptom associated with more than 60 different medical conditions. Low back pain can range from mild to severe discomfort. It may also radiate to the buttocks, hips, thighs and calves. Back pain may strike suddenly. Or, it may develop over a long period of time. There are two types:

- Acute back pain lasts from several days to a few weeks. It's often the result of an injury. Symptoms range from a dull muscle ache to shooting or stabbing pain that may decrease your flexibility and ability to move or stand up straight.
- Chronic back pain persists for more than three months. It may get worse with time.

Most cases of back pain are caused by mechanical disorders affecting the back and spine. Examples include herniated discs, muscle strains and osteoarthritis. But, low back pain also may be caused by other medical conditions and diseases. Endometriosis, fibromyalgia, infections and kidney stones are just a few examples. In addition, people with osteoporosis are particularly at risk of compression fractures.

DECIDING YOUR NEXT STEP

CALL 911:

- You have signs of shock. This may include a rapid heartbeat, rapid breathing, low blood pressure, faintness, confusion, lack of alertness, sweating, pale skin and a weak pulse.
- You're in severe pain, with sudden tearing or ripping pain that may radiate to the abdomen.
- You have sudden paralysis of your arms, legs or trunk.

SEEK EMERGENCY HELP:

- You have back pain after a new blow or fall.
- You become lightheaded or faint, lose bowel or bladder control, or experience shaking chills.
- You have new severe weakness, numbness or tingling in your arms, legs or torso.
- You're in severe pain.

SEE YOUR DOCTOR TODAY:

- You have localized back pain and a fever.
- You have intense pain that may move toward your groin.
- You're in pain and are nauseous or vomiting.

CALL YOUR DOCTOR OR NURSE HELP LINE:

- Your pain travels down your legs below the knee.
- You have weakness or numbness in your buttocks, groin, thighs or calves.
- Your pain gets worse when you lie down, or wakes you up at night.
- Your pain is limiting your activity level. It also may be affecting the way you walk.
- Your pain has lasted longer than two weeks, despite self-care.
- You're pregnant.
- You have osteoporosis, a history of cancer or a weakened immune system.

(Continued)

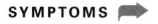
DECIDING YOUR NEXT STEP *(Continued)*
TRY SELF-CARE:
• You have pain, but without any of the symptoms above.

SMART ACTIONS TODAY
If your symptoms indicate self-care:

Ice it down. To help reduce pain and swelling, apply an ice pack, wrapped in a towel, to your back. A cold compress also will work. Hold it there for 10 to 15 minutes, three or four times per day, for the first 24 hours. If you have nerve damage, diabetes or poor circulation, check with your doctor first.

Then, turn up the heat. If pain persists after two days, apply heat—such as a heating pad—for brief periods. Or, take warm baths to relax your muscles and increase blood flow.

Try over-the-counter relief. Pain relievers, such as aspirin, naproxen and ibuprofen, may help reduce stiffness, swelling and inflammation. Follow the package directions carefully. Check with your doctor if you are pregnant or breast-feeding, or if you're not sure whether a certain medication is safe for you. *Caution:* Never give aspirin to anyone younger than age 19. It's linked to a rare but sometimes fatal condition called Reye's syndrome.

Work out the kinks. Physical activity, such as walking, may speed recovery. Start any exercise slowly, then increase activity as your pain improves. Ask your doctor or physical therapist for a list of gentle exercises to try.

SMART ACTIONS TOMORROW

Try these tips to help prevent repeated episodes of back pain:

Reduce your risk factors. Maintaining a healthful weight and quitting smoking are two ways to help your back. Both obesity and smoking are associated with a higher risk of back pain.

Sit right. Pick a chair with good back support. For additional comfort, place a small pillow or rolled-up towel behind the small of your back. This also works well in the car. Always try to sit with your shoulders back. Place a stool under your feet so that your knees are higher than your hips. Get up every hour to walk and stretch.

Stand smart. Stand with your head up, shoulders straight, chest forward and stomach tight.

Get sleep support. Choose a firm mattress and a box spring that doesn't sag. The best sleep position is on your side with your knees bent, with one pillow beneath your head and another between your knees.

Lifting Tips

Try to use a luggage cart or dolly to move heavy loads. If you must lift, stand with your feet wide apart and bend your knees. Don't bend at your waist. Tighten your stomach muscles as you lift. Keep your back as flat as possible. Don't arch, bend or twist. When carrying heavy items, hold them close to your body and centered, not off to one side. To slide heavy items, push them using your leg strength. Don't pull.

BONE INJURIES— EXTREMITIES

UNDERSTANDING YOUR SYMPTOMS

A broken bone always needs medical attention. That may seem obvious. But, unless you see a bone poking through your skin, you may not know if you've actually broken a bone. That's because the break could be very small, as with a stress fracture. Or, you could have chipped or shattered a bone. On occasion, bone breaks can't be seen immediately by X-ray. Other imaging tests or repeat X-rays may be needed later. Injuries aren't always breaks. For example, you may have a dislocation.

It's important to get medical help if you've had a bad fall or injury and think you've hurt a bone. Depending on your injury, moving when you have a bone or joint injury may cause more damage. Possible symptoms of a broken bone include a misshapen limb or joint, swelling or bruising, intense pain, an inability to move the injured area or bone sticking through broken skin. If you don't have any of the above symptoms, you still may have a fracture. Or, you may have a sprain or strain. See Sprains, Page 192.

---

56 ▶ ## DECIDING YOUR NEXT STEP

CALL 911:

- You've had a major fall, car accident or injury.
- You're bleeding severely.
- The area below the injury is cold, clammy, pale or blue. This could mean your circulation has been affected.
- Bone has broken through the skin.
- You're having trouble breathing.

- Your hurt limb is in an odd position or angle.
- You have signs of shock. This may include a rapid heartbeat, rapid breathing, low blood pressure, faintness, confusion, lack of alertness, sweating, pale skin and a weak pulse.

SEEK EMERGENCY HELP:
- You're in severe pain.
- You're unable to move, bear weight or use the bone.
- Your hurt finger or toe is in an odd position or angle.

SEE YOUR DOCTOR TODAY:
- You have rapid swelling, or bruising.
- You heard a pop or felt a snap when you were injured.
- You have osteoporosis or other bone disorder, or a bleeding disorder.
- You've had surgery or a previous fracture to the injured bone.

CALL YOUR DOCTOR OR NURSE HELP LINE:
- You have increased swelling, pain or bruising a day later.
- You don't feel any better after three days.

TRY SELF-CARE:
- Self-care is usually not appropriate for a bone injury.

SMART ACTIONS TODAY

Until you get emergency help. Apply pressure to a bleeding wound with a sterile bandage or cloth. Don't attempt to straighten the injured bone. If possible, stabilize it by making a splint with any available firm material.

SMART ACTIONS TOMORROW

To reduce your risk of injury, try these precautions:

Play smart and watch your step. Protective gear is a must for all athletic activities. Also, use a rubber mat in the tub. Use ladders or sturdy step stools when reaching.

BREATHING PROBLEMS

UNDERSTANDING YOUR SYMPTOMS

A stuffy nose is common with a cold or respiratory infection. See also Coughs, Page 114, or Nasal Congestion, Page 167. But, some conditions can lead to more serious breathing problems.

- Anaphylaxis is a life-threatening allergic reaction. Symptoms usually develop within seconds or minutes. But, sometimes they can occur hours later. You may have wheezing or difficulty breathing. If you have signs of a severe allergic reaction, call 911. Prompt emergency help is required.
- An asthma attack tightens and narrows the muscles around the airways to and from your lungs. It also causes the airway linings to swell.
- Chronic obstructive pulmonary disease (COPD) includes emphysema and chronic bronchitis. In emphysema, the walls between your lungs' air sacs have been damaged. In bronchitis, airways become narrow and inflamed. And, your lungs produce more mucus.
- Pulmonary embolism (PE), or a blood clot in the lung, lowers the flow of oxygen to the lung and other organs. It may result in death. Shortness of breath is one sign. But, sufferers often have no symptoms.

Trend Line

- 16.1 million American adults have asthma.
- 13.6 million American adults have COPD.

Source: National Center for Health Statistics

57 ▶ DECIDING YOUR NEXT STEP

CALL 911:

- You have severe difficulty breathing. Or, you make a loud, harsh croaking or crowing sound while breathing.
- You may be having an allergic reaction to something such as an insect sting, food or medication.
- You are choking or something is caught in your throat.
- You have chest pain, pressure, tightness, heaviness, indigestion or fatigue.
- Your throat is severely swollen.

SEEK EMERGENCY HELP:

- You have a fever of 104° F or higher.
- You have a history of blood clots, or you are pregnant or have had any of the following in the last four weeks: trauma, chemotherapy, hospitalization, childbirth or surgery. Or, you have been immobilized or were sitting for a lengthy period, such as on a long flight.

SEE YOUR DOCTOR TODAY:

- You have nonstop, continuous coughing.
- Your activities are limited because you feel winded.
- Your ankles are swollen and you're feeling breathless, especially upon exertion or when you're on your back.

CALL YOUR DOCTOR OR NURSE HELP LINE:

- You have difficulty breathing not described above.

TRY SELF-CARE:

- Self-care is not appropriate. Breathing difficulty requires medical evaluation.

SMART ACTIONS TODAY

If your symptoms indicate emergency care:

Stay calm. Panic increases breathing difficulty. Sit up if possible. Limit your activities.

If you're having an allergic reaction:

Use epinephrine, if prescribed. Follow the instructions in the epinephrine kit. Usually, the best injection site is the upper thigh. Call 911.

Remove insect stingers. Use a fingernail or credit card to scrape the stinger out of the skin. Be careful not to pinch it or push it farther in.

If you're having an asthma attack:

Use your rescue inhaler. This medicine should begin to open your airways in just minutes. Follow the emergency action plan as directed by your doctor.

MYTH OR TRUTH?

YOU CAN EXERCISE YOUR BREATHING

TRUTH. If you have COPD, ask your doctor about special retraining exercises. These can help you inhale and exhale with less difficulty.

SMART ACTIONS TOMORROW

Some steps to take to breathe easier:

Quit smoking. Steer clear of secondhand smoke, too. It may trigger asthma and aggravate COPD symptoms.

Prepare for allergies. If you know you're allergic to insect bites, foods or drugs, be prepared. Carry an emergency kit with injectable epinephrine and an antihistamine. Be sure you know how to use the kit. Also, wear a medical-alert bracelet.

Avoid triggers. Read food labels carefully. If you have a drug allergy, ask your doctor about other drugs in the same category that you also may need to avoid.

Control asthma. Work with your doctor to come up with a written action plan. Talk about whether you need long-term medicines. Ask how to prevent and treat flare-ups.

Avoid colds and the flu. Wash hands often with soap and warm water for 20 seconds. And, get a flu vaccine.

Breathe easier indoors. Rid your home of irritants such as dust, smoke, fumes and strong smells. Be sure your kitchen exhaust fan works. Use it as needed. If you have your home painted or exterminated, stay out of the house until the fumes clear. Open a door or window if you use a wood stove or kerosene heater. Keep doors and windows shut when outdoor pollution or pollen levels are high.

Get active. Regular exercise is good for your muscles, including those used to breathe. Always check with your doctor before starting an exercise program.

BRUISES

UNDERSTANDING YOUR SYMPTOMS

When you hurt the soft tissue under your skin, you may get a bruise. The swelling and black-and-blue color is a result of blood leaking from tiny blood vessels that have been damaged. Older adults bruise more easily because their blood vessels are more fragile. In general, bruises heal in one to four weeks. Most are caused by injuries. But, sometimes medications, an underlying illness or a medical condition is to blame. An infection, immune system disorder, or blood or blood vessel abnormalities are a few examples.

---

58 ➤ ## DECIDING YOUR NEXT STEP

SEEK EMERGENCY HELP:

- You've hurt your head and have bruising behind the ear or around both eyes.
- You have major or rapid swelling at the injury site and large or immediate black-and-blue marks.
- You have widespread bruising. You also have bleeding that you can't explain.

SEE YOUR DOCTOR TODAY:

- You're pregnant, have given birth, or had an abortion or miscarriage within the past six weeks, and have unexplained bruising.
- You've recently had a blood transfusion or surgery.
- You have a fever and multiple bruises.
- You have a weakened immune system, chronic medical condition, or a bleeding or clotting disorder. Or, you take a blood thinner, such as aspirin or warfarin (Coumadin).

CALL YOUR DOCTOR OR NURSE HELP LINE:
- You have swelling around the bruise, especially at a joint.
- Your bruise becomes firm or starts increasing in size.
- You weren't injured but have multiple bruises and possibly bleeding gums.

TRY SELF-CARE:
- Your bruise is small.

SMART ACTIONS TODAY

If your symptoms indicate self-care:

Raise and wrap. If possible, keep the bruised area above heart level after the injury. If swelling persists, loosely wrap the area with an elastic bandage or soft cloth.

Keep it cold. Wrap ice in a towel. Or, use a cold compress. Place it on the bruise for 10 to 15 minutes. Repeat three to four times a day for the first 24 hours. If you have nerve problems, diabetes or poor circulation, check with your doctor first.

Relieve the pain. You can take acetaminophen to help with minor pain. Follow the package directions carefully. Check with your doctor if you are pregnant or breast-feeding, or if you're not sure whether a certain medication is safe for you. Don't take aspirin or NSAIDs if you have bruises. They may slow blood clotting. They also can prolong bleeding under the skin.

SMART ACTIONS TOMORROW

If you have unexplained bruises, consider the following:

Your medication. Ask your doctor if your medication may be the cause. If it is, ask if there's an alternative. *Caution:* Never stop taking a prescription without your doctor's OK.

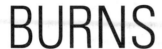

BURNS

UNDERSTANDING YOUR SYMPTOMS

A minor burn from an iron or a hot stove is painful. But, it's usually treatable at home. Other types and severities of burns, though, will require different levels of treatment. The types include thermal burns from fire, steam or liquids. Chemical burns, electrical burns and radiation burns are other types. Here's what you need to know about burns:

- First degree is when only the outer layer of skin is burned. You'll have pain and redness. This is known as a superficial epidermis burn.
- Second-degree burns—also called partial-thickness burns—involve the top two layers of skin. Pain is intense, and the skin is red, pink or white. Blisters may form.
- Third degree, or full thickness, is when *all* the underlying skin tissues are damaged. Sometimes, underlying structures may be burned, too. The skin is charred and leathery. There is severe swelling. And, if the nerve endings are destroyed, there may be no pain.
- Chemical burns, like thermal burns, may be first, second or third degree. And, depending on the chemical, they may cause other bodily damage if absorbed into the skin.
- Electrical burns are similarly unpredictable. Strong currents may cause internal damage you can't always see.
- Radiation burns occur after long stints in the sun or in a tanning bed, or as a side-effect of radiation treatments.

---

59 ⮞ ## DECIDING YOUR NEXT STEP
CALL 911:

- You have signs of shock. This may include a rapid heartbeat, rapid breathing, low blood pressure, faintness, confusion, lack of alertness, sweating, pale skin and a weak pulse.
- You have difficulty breathing or are wheezing.

- You have a burn to the eye.
- You've been struck by lightning.
- You've been in a fire and now have a headache, dizziness, nausea, sleepiness or confusion.
- You've been in a fire and burned the inside of your nose or mouth.
- Large parts of your body have been burned.
- You've been burned and the swelling is spreading rapidly.

SEEK EMERGENCY HELP:
- You have a second-degree burn that is larger than your palm or spread over large areas of a particular body part.
- You have a burn that's red, tender and blistered on a joint or on your face, hands, feet, groin, buttocks or skin folds.
- Your skin is leathery and white, black or brown.
- You've inhaled toxic fumes.
- You have any third-degree — or full-thickness — burn.
- You've received more than a minor electrical shock.

SEE YOUR DOCTOR TODAY:
- You have severe pain that's lasted for at least two hours, despite taking medication.
- You have increased redness, swelling, warmth or pus.
- You've been burned and have a weakened immune system or a chronic medical condition.

CALL YOUR DOCTOR OR NURSE HELP LINE:
- You're still in pain after 48 hours.
- Your burn doesn't heal in one week.
- You haven't had a tetanus shot within the past five years, you haven't completed the tetanus series, or you're not sure when you had your last tetanus shot.

TRY SELF-CARE:
- You have a minor burn with no other symptoms.

SMART ACTIONS TODAY

If your symptoms indicate emergency care:

Cool and cover. Drape a burn caused by heat with a moist, damp bandage or sterile cloth. Do this only if the burn area isn't large. Use a cool compress on an electrical burn.

Rinse off chemicals right away. For any chemical burn to the eye, flush with running water for 15 minutes or until help arrives. For liquid chemical burns to other areas, flush with water for 20 minutes. If the chemical was dry, first brush any remaining product off your skin. Then, flush as above. Keep the container or label to show to medical staff. Never use ointments or salves on chemical burns.

Take it off. If it can be done safely, remove belts and jewelry that might impede swelling. Remove clothing that may have been exposed to chemicals.

Get in position. If possible, elevate the affected area to reduce swelling. If shock seems possible, lie flat and elevate your feet about 12 inches. *Caution:* Never do this if the position causes pain—or if injuries to the head, neck, back or legs are suspected.

If your symptoms indicate self-care:

Cool down. Put the injured area under cool running water for at least 10 minutes. Or, immerse the burned area in cool water. Cool compresses also may be applied.

Change and clean daily. If the burn is blistered or open, apply an antibiotic ointment. Then, cover it with a clean bandage. Don't break blisters. They protect the area. At least once a day, gently clean the burn with mild soap and water. Then, reapply ointment and a fresh bandage.

Relieve pain. Take an over-the-counter pain reliever. Follow the package directions carefully. Check with your doctor if you are pregnant or breast-feeding, or if you're not sure whether a certain medication is safe for you. *Caution:* Never give aspirin to anyone younger than age 19. It's linked to a rare but sometimes fatal condition called Reye's syndrome.

MYTH OR TRUTH?

ICE IS NICE

MYTH. Icing a burn injury may cause frostbite. You also don't want to remove clothing that's stuck to burned skin. Blowing on or applying butter to a burn, and breaking blisters are other don'ts.

SMART ACTIONS TOMORROW

The Safe Tips chapter lists simple ways to reduce your risk of getting burned. See Page 66. Here are a few quick tips:

Guard against scalding. Keep your water heater at 120° F.

Cook safely. Don't wear loose clothing around the stove, and turn cookware handles toward the rear of the stove.

Take care with chemicals. Read and follow label instructions on all chemical products. Use paints, ammonia and other products that give off fumes in a well-ventilated area. Store flammable liquids in their original, clearly labeled containers. Keep them away from pilot lights and other sources of ignition.

Take care with cords. Replace worn or broken electrical cords. Also, don't hide cords beneath carpets. The cords may fray.

Arm the alarm. Check and change the batteries in your smoke alarms every six months.

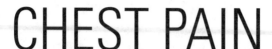

CHEST PAIN

UNDERSTANDING YOUR SYMPTOMS

While chest pain may be mild in nature—meaning it may not stop you in your tracks—it may signify a serious event. **That's why you should call 911 immediately if any of your symptoms indicate the possibility of a heart attack.**

There are many different signs of a heart attack. Severe chest pain is the most obvious one. But, there are several more subtle signs. This is especially true if you're a woman, you have diabetes or you're age 65 or older. These other symptoms include shortness of breath; pain in the upper back, neck, jaw or other areas of the upper body; nausea or vomiting; breaking out into a cold sweat; or lightheadedness.

Chest pain is any discomfort felt between your neck and your upper abdomen. But, this pain doesn't always mean you're having a heart attack. Here are other possible causes of heart-related chest pain:

- Aortic dissection causes sudden, searing pain between your shoulder blades. That's when the inner layers of the main artery leading away from your heart tear.
- Angina may feel like pressure or tightness in your chest. This is when blood flow to your heart is limited. A coronary artery spasm may be another reason for a tight feeling.
- Pericarditis may give you a sharp, knifelike pain over the center or left side of the chest. This is inflammation in the sac around your heart.

Other kinds of chest pain are unrelated to the heart:

- Costochondritis is a condition that causes a rib or rib cartilage to become inflamed. Your sternum and ribs will probably feel tender and sore under light pressure.
- Heartburn is a painful, burning sensation behind your lower breastbone. The feeling may last for hours.
- Muscle-related pain, typically, is felt only when you push on the area.

- Sharp pain that worsens when you take a deep breath or cough could be caused by pneumonia, pulmonary embolism (a blood clot in your lung), pneumothorax (the collapse of a small area of a lung) or pleurisy (an inflammation of the outer lung lining). This list does not include every possible cause for chest pain.

Don't Delay!

If your chest pain symptoms point to a heart attack, call 911 right away. Emergency medical services can start treatment as soon as they arrive. Don't try to diagnose chest pain yourself.

---

60 ▶ DECIDING YOUR NEXT STEP

CALL 911:

- You have chest pain that could be crushing, squeezing or severe, or feels like pressure or tightness. It lasts more than a few minutes or goes away and comes back.
- Your pain may be felt in or move to your neck, jaw, throat, back, shoulders, abdomen or arms.
- You feel sweaty, dizzy, lightheaded, nauseous, short of breath or are vomiting.
- You have a rapid or irregular heartbeat.
- You have angina, but the pain is more intense. Or, it's triggered by relatively light activity or while you're at rest.
- You have sudden, sharp chest pain with shortness of breath, especially after a long trip, a period of bed rest, or other lack of movement that may have led to a blood clot.
- You may not have chest pain, but you have persistent indigestion or fatigue.

(Continued)

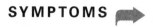

DECIDING YOUR NEXT STEP *(Continued)*

SEEK EMERGENCY HELP:

• You have a history of blood clots, or you are pregnant or have had any of the following in the last four weeks: trauma, chemotherapy, hospitalization, childbirth or surgery. Or, you have been immobilized or were sitting for a lengthy period, such as on a long flight.

SEE YOUR DOCTOR TODAY:

• You have chest pain with no known cause.

TRY SELF-CARE:

• You know that coughing, an injury or overexertion has caused muscle strain. Your chest wall is tender or painful when you press the area with your finger.

SMART ACTIONS TODAY

If your symptoms indicate self-care:

Ease the pain. If the cause of your chest pain is muscle strain, OTC pain relievers may help. Follow package directions carefully. Check with your doctor if you're pregnant or breast-feeding, or if you're not sure whether a certain medication is safe for you. You may also apply heat or an ice pack wrapped in a towel. Do this for 10 to 15 minutes. Repeat three to four times a day for the first 24 hours. If you have nerve damage, diabetes or poor circulation, check with your doctor first. Also, be sure to rest.

Follow doctor's orders. If the cause of your chest pain is previously diagnosed asthma or angina, follow your doctor's instructions. Take any prescribed medications.

SMART ACTIONS TOMORROW

The cause of your chest pain will determine what steps you may take to prevent a recurrence.

To help prevent heart attack and angina:

Know your risks. Evaluate your risk factors. Discuss them with your doctor. Risk factors for heart disease include a family history of early heart disease, high blood pressure and high cholesterol. Other factors are smoking, being overweight or obese, lack of exercise and having diabetes. Your risk also increases as you get older.

Follow a heart-healthy lifestyle. That includes maintaining a healthy weight. And, be sure to follow a diet low in fat and cholesterol. Include lots of whole grains, fruits and vegetables. With your doctor's OK, exercise for at least 30 minutes a day, five days a week. If you have diabetes, control your blood sugar. Keep blood pressure and cholesterol in check. If you smoke, quit. Try to avoid secondhand smoke, too. Avoid stress as much as possible. Finally, if you drink, keep alcohol use to a minimum. That means no more than one drink a day for women, two for men.

To prevent other chest pain-related conditions:

Know your history. For aortic dissection, try to find out if any family members have (or had, if deceased) this condition. Talk with your doctor about proper screenings, lifestyle changes and any treatments that are necessary.

Keep moving. When traveling or sitting for long periods of time, get up frequently and move around. This is to prevent pulmonary embolism. If you can't get up, at least flex your calf muscles and rotate your ankles to promote good circulation. Do this 10 times every 30 minutes.

COUGHS

UNDERSTANDING YOUR SYMPTOMS

Coughing is usually associated with a cold or upper respiratory infection. Allergies often lead to coughs, too. In both cases, the cough may be related to postnasal drip. If mucus reaches your airways, it may irritate them, leading to a cough. But, that's just one of several conditions that may cause a cough. Here are a few of the more common causes:

- Acute bronchitis is an infection of the lungs that's usually viral. It causes a cough that may be present for 10 days to two weeks. Mucus may be yellow, green, gray, brownish or white.
- Asthma may cause coughing and wheezing during an attack, or when the condition isn't well controlled.
- Chronic conditions such as chronic obstructive pulmonary disease (COPD) may lead to coughing.
- Lung cancer has many different symptoms. Cough, sometimes associated with bloody mucus, is a common symptom.
- Pneumonia, usually from an infection, occurs when the lungs are inflamed. Sufferers usually have cough, fever and sometimes trouble breathing.
- Cigarette smoke irritates your airways and harms cilia, the microscopic hairs that normally sweep debris from your airways. You cough as your airways try to keep themselves clean.
- Other causes of coughing include congestive heart failure, heartburn and tuberculosis. Sometimes, blood pressure medicines, such as angiotensin-converting enzyme (ACE) inhibitors, are the cause.

61 DECIDING YOUR NEXT STEP

CALL 911:
- You're coughing up a large amount of blood.
- You have chest pain, shortness of breath, persistent indigestion, or tightness or heaviness in the jaw, teeth, throat, arms, shoulders, back or upper abdomen.
- If you're wheezing or having difficulty breathing, see Breathing Problems, Page 100.

SEEK EMERGENCY HELP:
- You're coughing up bloody or pink-and-frothy matter.
- You have intense shaking chills—more than just shivering.
- You have a history of blood clots, or you are pregnant or have had any of the following in the last four weeks: trauma, chemotherapy, hospitalization, childbirth or surgery. Or, you've been immobilized or were sitting for a lengthy period, such as on a long flight.
- You have a fever of 104° F.

SEE YOUR DOCTOR TODAY:
- You have a fever and are pregnant.
- You're coughing up flecks of blood or rust-colored matter.
- You're coughing continuously. Or, you're coughing up colored sputum.
- You have a fever of 103° F or higher.

CALL YOUR DOCTOR OR NURSE HELP LINE:
- You have asthma and your cough is getting worse.
- You've had a fever of 101° F for 24 hours or longer.
- You've been taking an antibiotic for an upper respiratory infection for 48 hours with no improvement.
- You cough when you exercise.
- You've been coughing for more than three weeks or your cough is disrupting your daily activities.
- You have diabetes or a weakened immune system.

(Continued)

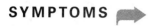
DECIDING YOUR NEXT STEP *(Continued)*
TRY SELF-CARE:
• You have a cough but none of the symptoms above.

SMART ACTIONS TODAY
If your symptoms indicate self-care:

Think twice about cough medicine. A productive cough is one of your body's ways of clearing infection and irritants from your airways. Therefore, talk with your doctor or pharmacist before using OTC cough medicine.

Rest right. Sleep can help your body fight an infection. If coughing disrupts your sleep, try using two pillows.

Turn up the moisture. A cool-mist humidifier will keep mucus membranes moist and less vulnerable to irritation. Clean it daily or as instructed by the manufacturer. Running a hot shower and inhaling the steam also may help.

Avoid smoke. It will irritate any kind of cough.

Drink liquids. This may help make mucus easier to cough up. Try warm drinks, such as tea with lemon and honey.

Treat asthma. Use your rescue inhaler. It should start to open your airways in a matter of minutes. Follow your emergency action plan. Just remember, your rescue inhaler is not a substitute for daily, long-term control medicines.

SMART ACTIONS TOMORROW

Avoid common cough triggers with these strategies:

Stop smoking. Smoking is the major cause of COPD, which is characterized by chronic coughing. Talk with your doctor about ways to quit.

Stay clean. Wash your hands often with soap and warm water, for 20 seconds. Do this especially if someone near you has a cold. Keep surfaces you touch clean. Alcohol-based wipes or gel sanitizers work, too.

Prevent flu. Get your annual flu shot or nasal vaccine. Ideally, you should do so six to eight weeks before flu season revs up. See Influenza, Page 148. A pneumonia shot is also available. Talk with your doctor to see if it's right for you.

Rule out gastroesophageal reflux. Sometimes, a stubborn cough is the only warning sign that stomach acids are backwashing into your esophagus. See your doctor for an evaluation that may help determine if this could be the cause.

Question your meds. About one in five people who take blood pressure-lowering ACE inhibitors develops a persistent dry cough. Ask your doctor if this might be causing your cough.

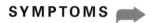

CUTS

UNDERSTANDING YOUR SYMPTOMS

A cut is any tear in the skin—straight or jagged. It may bleed, resulting in a scab. This acts as a germ barrier and allows the tissue underneath to heal. But, this natural healing process may get off track, especially if the wound isn't cared for properly. And, certain factors, such as aging, diabetes or a weakened immune system, also may make it more difficult for the body to mend itself.

---

62 ▶ **DECIDING YOUR NEXT STEP**

CALL 911:

- You have uncontrollable bleeding.
- You have a deep cut on your head, torso or neck.
- You have signs of shock. This may include a rapid heartbeat, rapid breathing, low blood pressure, faintness, confusion, lack of alertness, sweating, pale skin and a weak pulse.

SEEK EMERGENCY HELP:

- Your cut is jagged or large, or appears to be more than one-quarter inch deep.
- Your cut gets in the way of movement or function—as in the case of a wound to a joint.
- You've cut your eye, eyelid or lips.
- Your bleeding won't stop after 10 minutes of firm pressure.

SEE YOUR DOCTOR TODAY:

- You haven't had a tetanus shot within the past five years, you haven't completed the tetanus series, you're not sure when you had your last tetanus shot, or you have a weakened immune system.
- Your cut is on your face, ear or hand.
- You have an object or debris caught in the cut.

- Your stitches have become loose or the wound has separated or opened.
- You take a blood thinner or have a bleeding disorder.
- You have a rapidly spreading area around your cut that is red, swollen, hot and tender, or painful.
- You see red streaks or pus draining from the wound.

CALL YOUR DOCTOR OR NURSE HELP LINE:
- You're not sure if your cut may need stitches.

TRY SELF-CARE:
- You have a minor cut, with no other symptoms.

SMART ACTIONS TODAY

If your symptoms indicate emergency care:

Stop the bleeding. If possible, elevate the area that's bleeding to just above heart level. Cover it with a clean cloth. Apply direct pressure until emergency help arrives. If the cloth becomes soaked with blood, don't remove it. Put another cloth on top and continue to apply steady pressure.

If your wound doesn't require emergency care:

Wash wisely. After washing your hands well, run a steady stream of cool water over the injury. Then, clean the area with mild soap. Don't dig around in the wound.

Apply pressure. If your cut is still bleeding after it's been washed and dried, apply firm pressure with a sterile piece of gauze. Most cuts stop bleeding after a few minutes.

Guard against germs. Antibiotic creams may help guard against infections. Follow the directions carefully.

(Continued)

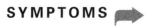
SMART ACTIONS TODAY *(Continued)*

Cover it up. An undressed wound will heal faster. But, if it's in an area where it may get dirty or irritated by clothing, it's best to cover the cut with an adhesive bandage. Change the bandage daily. Also, keep healing cuts out of the sun.

SMART ACTIONS TOMORROW

Taking simple precautions, such as handling sharp objects with care, will prevent lots of nicks and cuts. Here are a few ideas you may not have thought of:

Soften your skin. Supple skin is stronger and more resistant to injury than dry, fragile skin. Use moisturizing creams to hydrate your skin. Creams are more concentrated and contain less water than lotions.

Avoid tetanus. Tetanus, a potentially fatal bacteria, is most commonly associated with rusty objects. However, it also lives in soil, dust and even saliva. Any cut in the skin may invite tetanus. That's why it's important to get a tetanus booster shot every 10 years.

What's a Puncture Wound?

Small puncture wounds are caused by sharp objects literally poking a hole through the skin. They're quite common on feet, especially during the summer months when many people go barefoot. When things such as glass, needles, nails and even seashells pierce the skin, they may force dirt, skin and clothing into the wound. It's important to contact your doctor after getting a puncture wound. He or she will be able to determine what type of care you're going to need.

DENTAL PROBLEMS

UNDERSTANDING YOUR SYMPTOMS

Don't ignore an aching tooth or sore gums. Here are some common dental problems:

- Bad breath, known as halitosis, is due to not brushing and flossing every day. But, gingivitis or other gum diseases also may affect your breath.
- Dental traumas may happen when you bite down on something hard or if you get hit in the mouth. The result may be a broken, cracked or lost tooth.
- Gum pain is usually caused by an infection and inflammation of the gums, known as periodontal disease.
- Toothaches often stem from untreated tooth decay or an infection. Other causes include an impacted tooth, teeth grinding, an abnormal bite, aftereffects of dental procedures, and damage to the tooth or crown.

---

63 ▶ DECIDING YOUR NEXT STEP

CALL 911:

- You have a toothache along with chest pain, pressure or discomfort that may move to your neck, jaw, throat, back, shoulders, abdomen or arms. You may be having a heart attack. See Chest Pain, Page 110.

SEEK EMERGENCY HELP:

- You've injured your mouth and your teeth, jaw or gums hurt.
- Your mouth is bleeding severely.
- Your mouth, face or neck are extremely swollen.
- Your toothache or mouth pain is extreme.

(Continued)

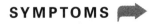

DECIDING YOUR NEXT STEP *(Continued)*

SEEK EMERGENCY HELP:

• You've just broken, visibly cracked or lost a tooth.

SEE YOUR DENTIST TODAY:

• You've had a tooth pulled and it's bled for four hours.
• You suddenly have severe pain after having had a tooth pulled at least 24 hours ago. Pain medicine doesn't help.
• You've lost a filling.
• You have a broken or cracked tooth that is sensitive to hot or cold temperatures or air.
• Your face or cheek is swollen.

CALL YOUR DENTIST OR NURSE HELP LINE:

• You have a toothache.
• Your toothache or gum pain gets worse.
• You're in pain following a dental procedure.
• You have tooth or mouth pain when eating or drinking—either hot or cold foods or beverages.
• Your tooth, a filling or a crown feels loose.
• You see a small chip or small crack in your tooth.
• You have constant bad breath combined with another ailment, such as a respiratory tract infection, chronic sinusitis, postnasal drip, chronic bronchitis, diabetes, stomach problems, or a liver or kidney illness. Your bad breath may be a symptom of your other condition.
• You have a sore or lump on your tongue, cheeks, lips or gums that's still there after two weeks.
• Your mouth is bleeding.
• You've tried self-care but it didn't work.

TRY SELF-CARE:

• Your toothache or gum discomfort is minor and no other symptoms are present.

SMART ACTIONS TODAY

If your symptoms indicate emergency care:

Take care of the tooth. If a tooth is knocked out, hold it by the crown and very gently rinse off the root with water. If you can, gently reinsert and hold the tooth in its socket. If that's not possible, put the tooth in a cup of milk or place it in your mouth between your cheek and gum and, without delay, bring it with you to the dentist.

If your symptoms indicate self-care:

Ease the pain. Aspirin, acetaminophen, ibuprofen or naproxen may help the pain. Follow the package directions carefully. Check with your doctor if you are pregnant or breast-feeding, or if you're not sure whether a certain medication is safe for you. *Caution:* Never give aspirin to anyone younger than age 19. It's linked to a rare but sometimes fatal condition called Reye's syndrome.

Prop up. Tooth pain may feel worse when you lie down, due to increased circulation to your head. When you go to bed, elevate your head with pillows.

MYTH OR TRUTH?

RUB ASPIRIN ON YOUR GUMS

MYTH. You may have heard that rubbing aspirin on the gums near an aching tooth relieves the pain. Don't do it! Rubbing aspirin or any other painkiller on your gums may burn the tissue. Instead, consider trying an over-the-counter topical anesthetic to temporarily numb the area and reduce discomfort. Follow the package directions. See your dentist for follow-up care as soon as possible.

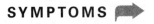

SMART ACTIONS TOMORROW

Research indicates that there may be a connection between advanced gum disease—known as periodontitis—and overall health problems, such as heart disease, stroke, diabetes and pneumonia. Here's how to keep your teeth and gums healthy:

Eat right. Follow a healthful diet that's low in sugar.

Brush at least twice a day. Use a soft toothbrush with fluoride toothpaste. Floss between teeth daily and gently brush your gums. Keep your bridge or dentures clean.

Write it down. Some medications may contribute to bad breath. Keep a log of the medications you take. Include over-the-counter medications, supplements and herbals. Also, let your dentist know if you've had any surgery, illness or change in your health since your last appointment.

Keep them clean. Have your teeth cleaned by a dentist or dental hygienist twice a year. This has been shown to prevent both decay and gum disease.

Stay safe. Wear a mouth guard and headgear while playing sports to help prevent mouth and teeth injuries.

Don't smoke or use tobacco in any form. Smoking or chewing tobacco may make some dental conditions worse, including gum disease, bad breath and dry mouth. They also may increase your risk of developing oral cancer.

DEPRESSION

UNDERSTANDING YOUR SYMPTOMS

Depression may take many forms. For some people, it's brought on by seasonal changes. For others, medications may be the cause. Chemical disorders, underlying medical conditions or life circumstances also may lead to depression. For some people, depression may be mild. For others, long-term feelings of sadness interfere with daily life.

  In any form, depression is a serious, but treatable, medical condition. And, it affects both the body and mind. One of the first steps toward treatment is identifying the type of depression you have. Here are the most common forms:

- Bipolar disorder, once known as manic-depressive illness, can consist of intense episodes of elation and/or despair. There also may be any combination of moods in between.
- Major depression involves symptoms that get in the way of daily activities such as eating, sleeping and work. You may lose interest in things you used to enjoy. Symptoms of major depression last for at least two weeks.
- Mild depression is also called dysthymia or dysthymic disorder. It's marked by general negativity, low energy, and feelings of hopelessness or dissatisfaction. Symptoms are less severe than those of major depression. But, they last much longer—for at least two years. Some people may suffer from both mild and major depression.
- Postpartum depression (PPD) sets in within a month of giving birth. Its symptoms are longer lasting and more severe than typical "baby blues." Those with a history of major depression are at a higher risk for PPD.
- Premenstrual dysphoric disorder (PMDD) consists of severe depression, tension and irritability. It typically sets in 10 to 14 days before the start of a menstrual cycle.
- Seasonal affective disorder (SAD) is depression that occurs in response to less daylight during the winter months.

64 ➤ DECIDING YOUR NEXT STEP

CALL 911:
- You're thinking of committing suicide.
- You're planning to harm someone.
- You're extremely confused or agitated.

SEEK EMERGENCY HELP:
- You're hallucinating. Or, you feel others are trying to hurt you.

SEE YOUR DOCTOR TODAY:
- You feel out of control.
- You're depressed after starting a new medication.

CALL YOUR DOCTOR OR NURSE HELP LINE:
- You're depressed after a major life change—such as job loss, childbirth, illness, divorce or the death of a loved one.
- You've started feeling anxious or depressed. Or, you've become restless, irritated or easily annoyed.
- Your symptoms continue or get worse despite treatment.

TRY SELF-CARE:
- You're feeling sad, with none of the above symptoms.

Trend Line

Depression affects an estimated 17 to 19 million Americans each year. Eighty percent of people who seek treatment experience improvement. While untreated depression puts you at risk of suicide, the earlier you get help, the sooner you'll be on track to feeling better.

Sources: Mental Health America and the National Women's Health Resource Center

SMART ACTIONS TODAY

Until you can get emergency care:

Dial for support. The National Suicide Prevention Lifeline operates a toll-free, 24-hour hotline at 1-800-273-TALK (1-800-273-8255). They have trained staff who can speak with you about what you're going through until help arrives.

Don't be alone. If you're having thoughts of suicide and are waiting for emergency help to respond, you should not be alone. Ask a family member or friend to stay with you until help arrives. Never drive yourself in this condition.

MYTH OR TRUTH?

DEPRESSION IS JUST A MENTAL CONDITION

MYTH. Some people with depression have an imbalance of brain chemicals called neurotransmitters. Aside from emotions, depression may have adverse effects on blood pressure, blood clotting, blood vessels, heart rhythms and the immune system.

SMART ACTIONS TOMORROW

Some self-help strategies to help you cope with depression:

Be patient. Depression won't disappear overnight. It may take three weeks or more for antidepressants to kick in or for depression to start to ease up with psychotherapy.

Stay away from substances. Don't reach for illicit drugs or alcohol when you're feeling blue. These things will only make your depression worse. Plus, they may cause dangerous side effects when taken with antidepressant medications.

(Continued)

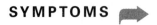

SMART ACTIONS TOMORROW (*Continued*)

Try to think positively. You might feel guilty. You may blame yourself for things you can't control. Or, you may expect to fail. Try to push these thoughts out of your mind. Learning how to think in a positive way may help ease your symptoms. Try to be an optimistic, helpful friend to *yourself*.

Reach out to others. Go out and take part in activities you enjoy. Have lunch with a friend. Go for a walk in the park. See a movie or play golf. Try activities that will make you feel good and give you a sense of accomplishment. Social support is critically important. Reach out to family members, friends and coworkers.

Put big decisions on hold. When you're feeling down, avoid making big life decisions. Now's not the best time to buy a house or change jobs, for example. If you find yourself faced with a major life decision, discuss it with someone you trust who will have a more objective point of view.

Get going. Exercise raises levels of feel-good hormones in your brain. Yoga, in particular, has the added benefit of helping you turn off your external surroundings. It can help you focus inward and think positive thoughts. Aim for at least 30 minutes of exercise per day, most days of the week. Check with your doctor before starting any exercise program.

Seek support. Simply talking with people who share problems similar to yours may do wonders. Look for a hospital- or community health-sponsored support group that focuses on a specific issue in your life, such as alcohol abuse or weight issues. Or, look for a self-help group without a specific theme.

DIZZINESS

UNDERSTANDING YOUR SYMPTOMS

Dizziness is a feeling of whirling, lightheadedness or unsteadiness. People sometimes say it feels as if they're about to fall. An occasional dizzy spell is usually caused by something minor. It may be due to an inner-ear infection, hyperventilation, motion sickness, overexertion in the heat or not eating. But, it also may be caused by a sudden drop in your blood pressure. This can happen if you've lost a lot of blood or if you're dehydrated.

If you feel that either you or your surroundings are moving, you may have a specific kind of dizziness called vertigo. There are many causes of vertigo. They include a stroke or tumor, inner-ear problems, low blood sugar and many more. The cause may be hard to pinpoint.

---

65 ▷ DECIDING YOUR NEXT STEP

CALL 911:

- You're experiencing a sudden onset of the following symptoms, which may indicate a stroke: numbness or weakness, especially in your face, arms or legs; trouble with your balance or coordination; difficulty with speaking or understanding other people's speech; confusion; trouble seeing in one or both eyes.
- You have chest pain or pressure. You also may have nausea, heart palpitations, or an irregular or rapid heartbeat. See Chest Pain, Page 110, for other possible signs of a heart attack.
- Your dizziness comes after exposure to a possible allergen, such as food, medicine or an insect sting.
- You recently ingested something toxic or poisonous.
- You have an excruciating headache.

(Continued)

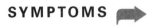

DECIDING YOUR NEXT STEP *(Continued)*

SEEK EMERGENCY HELP:

- You're severely dehydrated, with extreme thirst or decreased urine output. You may feel faint when you stand.
- You've had a head injury within the last three days.

SEE YOUR DOCTOR TODAY:

- You're dizzy and have an earache, ringing in the ear or hearing loss.
- You've had a head injury within the past month. Now, you're dizzy.
- You're moderately dehydrated, with moderate thirst and infrequent urination. And, your urine is dark yellow or amber.
- You have a fever or are nauseous and vomiting.

CALL YOUR DOCTOR OR NURSE HELP LINE:

- You're pregnant.
- You're age 65 or older and have a sudden onset of dizziness.
- You have a weakened immune system or a chronic medical condition, such as diabetes.
- You recently had surgery or were hospitalized.
- You're dizzy after starting a new prescription or over-the-counter medication.
- You're suddenly dizzy when you move your head a certain way.
- You've tried self-care, but it didn't stop your dizziness.
- You have unexplained dizziness.

TRY SELF-CARE:

- You know you're dizzy due to motion sickness.

SMART ACTIONS TODAY

If your symptoms indicate emergency care:

For those with diabetes. Check your blood sugar. Treat as needed.

SMART ACTIONS TOMORROW

Dizziness may be brought on by a number of medical conditions. Or, it may simply occur as a result of the way you move your body. These tips may help:

Take it slow. Try to remain quiet, or lie down, as you wait for the spell to pass. Once it does, move about carefully. Get up from a lying or sitting position slowly. Don't make sudden head movements. And, don't look up or down. Use extreme care with stairs.

Don't drive. It isn't safe to drive when you have dizziness. If you need to seek medical attention, have someone else drive you.

Fix what ails you. Ear infections, which may be caused by germs, are a main cause of dizziness in many people. Try to prevent them by frequently washing your hands with soap and warm water, for 20 seconds.

Stay well-hydrated. Drink enough water to stay hydrated throughout the day. This is especially important if you're sick.

Prevent motion sickness. If your dizziness is due to motion sickness, ask your doctor or pharmacist about over-the-counter medications. For other ways to deal with motion sickness, see Page 173.

EAR PROBLEMS

UNDERSTANDING YOUR SYMPTOMS

Ear problems range from itchiness and dull, aching pain to ringing and other noises in your ears. Some problems, such as swimmer's ear, are often related to a specific incident. Others, such as ringing, may be chronic and harder to treat. Here are some typical ear problems:

- Barotrauma happens when there's a sudden rise or fall in air pressure. This can be caused by airplane travel or scuba diving. Symptoms usually include ear pain and muffled hearing.

- A middle ear infection develops when the eustachian tubes become blocked. This is usually due to a cold, sinus infection or allergies. The fluid buildup may encourage infection. Symptoms include ear pain, fever and hearing loss. And, there may be a feeling of fullness in the ear as mucus builds up behind your eardrum. If your eardrum bursts, you may feel less pain and notice blood or pus draining from your ear.

- Swimmer's ear is an infection of the lining of the outer ear and ear canal. It's often caused by exposure to water contaminated with a certain germ. Other causes include scratching the ear canal or having an object stuck in your ear. Intense itching, redness and inflammation of the ear are usually the first signs. As the infection progresses, you may have pain that gets worse when you touch or pull on your outer ear.

- Tinnitus is a constant or occasional ringing, buzzing, whistling, hissing or roaring in your ears. This annoying and distracting noise is often associated with hearing loss or other medical problems.

DECIDING YOUR NEXT STEP

SEEK EMERGENCY HELP:

- You've recently injured your head or ear.
- You have a foreign object stuck in your ear.
- You have a fever of 104° F or higher.
- Your pain is severe, or you're severely ill.
- You have pain, swelling and redness behind the ear(s).
- You're dizzy or having trouble balancing.
- Your ear has been bleeding for at least 10 minutes.

SEE YOUR DOCTOR TODAY:

- You're pregnant and have a fever.
- You have a fever of 103° F or higher and your pain hasn't responded to treatment.
- You have diabetes or a weakened immune system.

CALL YOUR DOCTOR OR NURSE HELP LINE:

- You've had a fever of 101° F or higher for 24 hours.
- Your outer ear is swollen, red and itchy. Or, the pain gets worse when you touch your ear.
- Your ear has a yellow, sticky, bad-smelling discharge.
- You have tinnitus.
- You've been taking antibiotics for 48 hours with no improvement.
- Your hearing is muffled, or you've lost your hearing.

TRY SELF-CARE:

- You have none of the symptoms above.

Trend Line

An estimated 36 million Americans experience some tinnitus. More than 7 million say it interferes with daily life.

Source: American Academy of Otolaryngology, Head and Neck Surgery

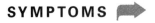

SMART ACTIONS TODAY

If your symptoms indicate self-care:

Apply gentle heat. Warm, moist heat may ease ear pain. Soak a clean washcloth in warm water. Hold it against the affected ear.

SMART ACTIONS TOMORROW

Here are some strategies to help you keep your ears healthy and pain-free:

Don't poke. Never stick anything in your ear canal, including cotton swabs. A cotton swab should be used only on your outer ear. Poking in the ear may pack earwax deep into your ear canal. It may also irritate the lining or injure your eardrum.

Sidestep plane pain. When on an airplane, don't sleep during the flight's descent. Suck on candy, chew gum or yawn frequently. This will keep your eustachian tubes open and relieve pressure in your ears. (Don't give gum or hard candy to children ages 4 and younger. It can cause choking.) Also, if you're planning a trip by airplane and are feeling congested or are already experiencing ear pain, speak with your doctor for advice before you fly.

Keep ears dry. If you're prone to swimmer's ear, wear earplugs when you swim, if directed by your doctor. And, never swim in polluted water. Don't let water run into your ears while bathing or washing your hair. Carefully dry your ears after swimming or bathing.

Guard against swimmer's ear. If you don't have a known hole in your eardrum, mix equal parts of white vinegar and water. Use a dropper to put a few drops into each ear after swimming. This helps kill germs that may lead to swimmer's ear.

Use protection. Noise may put your hearing at risk. Try to avoid exposure to loud noises. However, sometimes noise is nearly impossible to avoid, such as when operating a lawn mower or power tools. In these cases, wear earplugs or earmuffs. When using a portable listening device, such as a pocket music player or cell phone, keep the volume low—no more than 60 percent of its maximum. Keep it even lower if you're planning to use it for more than an hour. As a general rule, if you need to remove your headset to hear someone talking who's standing an arm's length away, your volume is turned up too loud.

Dive slowly. When scuba diving, descend and ascend slowly. And, don't dive if you're congested or suffering from allergies or a cold.

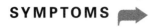

FAINTING

UNDERSTANDING YOUR SYMPTOMS

Fainting, also known as syncope, is a brief loss of consciousness. You may lose consciousness for about a minute. But, you usually recover quickly. Fainting occurs because there isn't enough oxygen getting to the brain.

There are many reasons for fainting. One of the most common reasons is because your nervous system is responding to pain, trauma or a sudden emotional upset, such as the sight of blood. Anemia, dehydration, standing in one position for too long and getting up too quickly are other reasons. And, certain blood pressure or heart medications also may lead to fainting. Other serious causes include pulmonary embolism, blood loss, arrhythmia, seizures, or cardiac or cerebral vascular disease.

---

67 ▷ DECIDING YOUR NEXT STEP

CALL 911:

- You're having trouble breathing. Or, you feel weak or have a rapid or irregular heartbeat.
- You have abdominal or chest pain or a severe headache.
- You were unconscious for longer than one minute.
- You are faint after exposure to a possible allergen. This includes food, medicine or an insect sting.
- You have signs of shock. This may include a rapid heartbeat, rapid breathing, low blood pressure, faintness, confusion, lack of alertness, sweating, pale skin and a weak pulse.
- You have a pacemaker or internal cardioverter defibrillator.

- You're experiencing a sudden onset of the following symptoms, which may indicate a stroke: Numbness or weakness, especially in your face, arms or legs; trouble with your balance or coordination; difficulty with speaking or understanding other people's speech; confusion; trouble seeing in one or both eyes.

SEEK EMERGENCY HELP:

- You fainted during exercise—or almost did. This includes feeling lightheaded or nauseous, or experiencing dimming of your vision or ringing in your ears.
- You fainted twice or more in one day—or almost did (see above).
- You have diabetes or are age 65 or older, weak or frail.
- You have felt near faint for longer than one hour.
- You have a history of heart disease or high blood pressure.
- You're severely dehydrated, with extreme thirst or decreased urine output. You may feel faint or dizzy when you stand. You may or may not have fainted.

SEE YOUR DOCTOR TODAY:

- You have an eating disorder.
- You've been on a diet.

CALL YOUR DOCTOR OR NURSE HELP LINE:

- You're pregnant or have a chronic medical condition.
- You fainted—or almost did—while coughing, stretching or going to the bathroom.
- You started a new over-the-counter or prescription medication.

TRY SELF-CARE:

- You fainted only once, were unconscious for less than a minute and your fainting was triggered by a stressful event. And, you didn't hurt yourself.

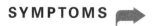
SMART ACTIONS TODAY

If your symptoms indicate emergency care:

For those with diabetes. Check your blood sugar and treat as needed.

If your symptoms indicate self-care:

Lie down. Lie with your head flat and your feet slightly elevated, 6 to 8 inches, to promote circulation. Loosen tight clothing.

Cool down. Drink some water or fruit juice. Place a cold washcloth on your forehead. Remain still for at least 30 minutes.

Get up slowly. And, sit for a few moments before you try to stand.

Write it down. Record everything you or a witness remembers about your fainting spell. Include the time, what you were doing and whether you were sitting or standing. Also, note any symptoms before, during or upon regaining consciousness. Then, share this information with your doctor.

MYTH OR TRUTH?

STAND STRAIGHT AND YOU MAY FAINT
TRUTH. Standing still for a long time may cause your blood to pool in your legs. This is especially true at times of emotional stress or during a heat wave. Keeping your knees locked may accelerate the process. Try to move around. Or, contract your leg muscles to keep your blood circulating. This will help keep you from fainting.

SMART ACTIONS TOMORROW

Follow these tips to help avoid future episodes of fainting:

Lie down. Do so after taking any prescribed medicine that causes you to feel faint.

Drink up. Drink enough fluids to stay hydrated. This is very important if you have a cold or other viral illness. However, if your doctor has limited fluids in your diet, follow his or her guidelines.

Move around. Avoid standing in one position for a long time. Shift your weight from foot to foot. Walk around whenever possible. And, men should sit down while urinating if they've ever fainted while standing up.

Don't drink alcohol. It tends to cause you to lose body fluids. It also lowers your blood pressure. That may make you more likely to faint.

Watch your blood sugar. If you have diabetes, always carry glucose tablets or hard candy. Your doctor may talk with you about an injection called glucagon for episodes of low blood sugar.

Exercise your legs. Do this especially if you're prone to fainting. Toned muscles may help move blood from the legs back to the heart. That may keep your blood pressure from dropping.

FEVERS

UNDERSTANDING YOUR SYMPTOMS

A fever is defined for adults as an ear or rectal temperature of more than 100.4° F, or an oral temperature of more than 99.5° F. Fever is usually your body's natural response to an infection or inflammation. It plays an important role in your body's defense against these two things. Everyone responds differently to infection and inflammation. So, the degree of your fever doesn't necessarily indicate the seriousness of your condition.

Most fevers run their course in two or three days. But, they may be the result of a range of conditions. Infections, problems with your immune system and even prolonged heat exposure could cause fever. Watch out for these possible conditions that can occur with fever:

- Dehydration may occur. That's because your body uses more fluids when you have a fever. Drinking enough water or other clear liquids to stay hydrated will help prevent this.

- Shivering usually occurs as your body temperature rises. It could occur once, or repeatedly. It could last a few minutes to an hour each time. True shaking chills, or rigors, are more intense and sudden than shivering. They may be a sign of a serious infection.

- Increased heart rate may occur as your temperature rises. Though, there are times when your heart rate may be lower than normal.

For most healthy adults, a fever may not need to be treated unless it's very high. This is not the case if you're pregnant, age 65 or older, have a weakened immune system or have heart or lung disease.

68 DECIDING YOUR NEXT STEP

CALL 911:

- You have faintness, confusion, lethargy, extreme weakness, or a rapid, weak pulse.
- You develop widespread bruising or a purplish, pinpoint rash that doesn't lose its color when pressed. This may indicate a clotting problem or body-wide infection.
- If you're wheezing or have severe difficulty breathing, see Breathing Problems, Page 100.

SEEK EMERGENCY HELP:

- You're severely dehydrated, with extreme thirst or decreased urine output. You may feel dizzy or faint when you stand.
- You have intense shaking chills—more than just shivering.

SEE YOUR DOCTOR TODAY:

- You're moderately dehydrated, with moderate thirst and infrequent urination. And, your urine may be dark yellow or amber.
- You have diabetes or a weakened immune system.
- You are pregnant, have given birth, or had an abortion or miscarriage within the past six weeks.
- You currently receive intravenous medications. Or, you use intravenous drugs.

CALL YOUR DOCTOR OR NURSE HELP LINE:

- You've had a fever for three days or longer.
- Your fever returns repeatedly without any known cause.
- You're age 65 or older.
- You have heart or lung disease.
- You've been hospitalized, been on prolonged bed rest, or had surgery or dental work within the past six weeks.
- You've been taking an antibiotic for two days or more and still have a fever.

(Continued)

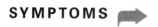

DECIDING YOUR NEXT STEP *(Continued)*

CALL YOUR DOCTOR OR NURSE HELP LINE:

- You've been taking a new prescription or over-the-counter (OTC) medication.
- You experience night sweats.
- You've recently traveled internationally.
- You have a prosthetic valve or joint.

TRY SELF-CARE:

- You have a mild, short-term fever and none of the symptoms above.

SMART ACTIONS TODAY

If your symptoms indicate self-care:

Reduce the fever. Try OTC pain relievers to reduce a fever of 102° F or higher. Follow the package directions carefully. Check with your doctor if you are pregnant or breast-feeding, or if you're not sure whether a certain medication is safe for you. *Caution:* Never give aspirin to anyone younger than age 19. It's linked to a rare but sometimes fatal condition called Reye's syndrome. If you're taking an OTC cough or cold medicine, check the ingredients to see if it also contains a fever reducer, so that you don't double dose.

Keep it light. Change into lightweight clothes. If you're shivering or cold, however, heavier clothing or blankets are fine until you feel warmer. Shivering causes your temperature to rise.

Sponge off. Wipe your body with a wet washcloth or take a lukewarm shower. Avoid cold water. And, don't use rubbing alcohol. These may cause shivering, which may raise your temperature.

Stay hydrated. Drink enough fluids to stay hydrated. Sip water and clear fruit juices. Snack on gelatin. Or, suck ice pops or ice chips. Don't drink alcohol.

SMART ACTIONS TOMORROW

Fevers are often caused by viral infections. Here are some tips to help you stay healthy:

Kill germs. Wash your hands often with soap and warm water, for 20 seconds. If you're not near a sink, use alcohol-based hand wipes or gels. Keep surfaces such as sinks, countertops, doorknobs and phones clean.

Get an annual flu vaccine. Ideally, try to get the vaccine six weeks before flu season begins. Ask your doctor which version—shot or nasal spray—is right for you. See Influenza, Page 148.

Boost immunity. Your body's immune system is your best defense against infections that cause fever. Protect it by eating well, exercising regularly and getting enough sleep.

MYTH OR TRUTH?

ALL THERMOMETERS ARE THE SAME

MYTH. They work in different ways. Here's what you need to know:

- A glass thermometer is no longer recommended due to concerns about mercury exposure.
- Digital thermometers provide quick, accurate readings.
- Ear thermometers are effective. But, they may be hard to use correctly. Also, readings may be inaccurate due to earwax.
- Skin thermometers are unreliable.

HEADACHES

UNDERSTANDING YOUR SYMPTOMS

Headaches come in many forms. They may be the pounding, jaw-clenching kind. Or, they may be simply an overall dull ache. The most common headache types are:

- Cluster: intense, steady pain that often occurs behind one eye, above one eye, or in the temple area. Clusters may recur several times a day. But, there may be symptom-free periods.
- Migraine: severe, often disabling pain, which is frequently accompanied by nausea, vomiting, and an aversion to bright light and noise. Migraine headaches typically are felt on one side of the head. They have a pulsating quality. Migraines generally last between four and 72 hours.
- Tension: the most common type of headache. Tension headaches are usually triggered by stress, poor posture or eyestrain.

Medical conditions, such as meningitis, tumors, hypertension, glaucoma, and sinus or viral infections, may cause what's known as a secondary headache.

Trend Line

An estimated 29.5 million Americans suffer from migraines. That number breaks down to about 6 percent of men and 18 percent of women. As many as 78 percent get tension headaches. Just 1 percent suffer from cluster headaches. These are primarily men.

Sources: National Headache Foundation and American Headache Society

69 DECIDING YOUR NEXT STEP

CALL 911:

- You suddenly get a headache that nearly disables you. You might describe it as the worst pain you've ever felt.
- You're experiencing a sudden onset of the following symptoms, which may indicate a stroke: Numbness or weakness, especially in your face, arms or legs; trouble with your balance or coordination; difficulty with speaking or understanding other people's speech; confusion; trouble seeing in one or both eyes.
- You become extremely ill. And, you develop a purplish, pinpoint rash or scattered, unusual bruising.

SEEK EMERGENCY HELP:

- You have a fever and feel severe neck pain or stiffness when you try to place your chin on your chest.
- You have a fever of 104° F or higher.
- You have severe eye pain. Or, your pupils become unequal in size.
- You have a severe headache that doesn't respond to pain relievers.

SEE YOUR DOCTOR TODAY:

- You have a headache combined with persistent nausea or vomiting.
- You're age 50 or older and have a headache combined with a sore scalp or pain around your temples.
- You have a weakened immune system.

CALL YOUR DOCTOR OR NURSE HELP LINE:

- Your headache keeps you from going about your daily activities. Pain relievers don't help.
- You've had a constant headache for more than two days.
- You get a headache after taking a new medication, including birth control pills.

(Continued)

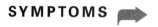

DECIDING YOUR NEXT STEP *(Continued)*

CALL YOUR DOCTOR OR NURSE HELP LINE:

- You notice a change in your typical headaches. For instance, your headaches get longer. Perhaps they're more severe or move to a different spot in your head.
- You get a headache during or right after strenuous activity—such as exercise, sexual intercourse, coughing, bending, lifting, sneezing, laughing or a bowel movement.
- You have frequent or persistent headaches.

TRY SELF-CARE:

- Your headache is mild, with none of the symptoms above.
- You get a headache after eating certain foods—such as foods with high MSG. Or, it hits after you drink alcohol or suddenly stop caffeine use.

SMART ACTIONS TODAY

If your symptoms indicate self-care:

Try a compress and stay hydrated. Soak a washcloth in cold water. Place it on your forehead or neck to soothe your aching head. Or, try moist heat in the form of a compress or hot shower. Rest in a quiet, darkened room. Drink enough liquids to stay hydrated.

Give it a rub. Massaging your neck and shoulder muscles may release some of the headache tension.

SMART ACTIONS TOMORROW

Some tips to help prevent headaches:

Get your rest. Poor sleep habits are a common cause of headaches. Get at least six to eight hours of sleep each night. Avoid sleeping in on the weekends. Try to go to bed and wake up at the same time each day.

Don't skip meals. This may lead to low blood sugar—a headache trigger.

Exercise regularly. With your doctor's OK, do moderate exercise three to five times a week. This may help reduce the frequency or severity of your headaches. But, don't exercise to the point of exhaustion. Also, keep your workout schedule steady. Inconsistent activity may actually trigger a headache.

Consider the caffeine connection. Sudden caffeine withdrawal is a frequent cause of headaches for some people.

De-stress. Stress causes your muscles to contract. This may lead to tension headaches. It also may cause you to turn to unhealthy coping strategies. See also Less Stress, Page 36.

Forego trigger foods. Different foods may trigger headaches in some people. Common triggers include red wine, beer, nuts, chocolate, aged cheeses and foods with MSG. Keep a food diary for a few weeks. It may help you spot a pattern. Note what you ate and when. Also, note how you felt in the hours that followed.

See your doctor. Migraine suffers may find relief from prescription medications, such as triptans. These are taken at the first sign of an attack. If you have migraines often, there are preventive medications you may be able to take. Talk with your doctor about all of the options.

MYTH OR TRUTH?

HEADACHES ARE A FACT OF LIFE

MYTH. Although some people are more prone to headaches than others, chronic, persistent headaches are not normal for anyone. If you suffer from headaches on a regular basis, see your doctor.

INFLUENZA

UNDERSTANDING YOUR SYMPTOMS

You ache all over. You're running a fever. You have a sore throat. And, you can barely pull yourself out of bed. You may have the flu. This contagious respiratory infection is brought on by influenza viruses. Every year, these easily spread viruses keep up to 20 percent of Americans off their feet for a week or so. The usual symptoms include body aches, extreme fatigue, headache, high fever and sore throat.

The infection may spread before symptoms appear. So, people may pass on the virus before they know they're sick. The flu season begins as early as October and usually peaks in January or later. New virus strains appear all the time. That's why new forms of vaccines are created each year.

---

70 ▷ ## DECIDING YOUR NEXT STEP

CALL 911:

- You have signs of shock. This may include a rapid heartbeat, rapid breathing, low blood pressure, faintness, confusion, lack of alertness, sweating, pale skin and a weak pulse.
- If you're wheezing or having severe difficulty breathing, see Breathing Problems, Page 100.

SEEK EMERGENCY HELP:

- You have a fever of 104° F or higher.
- You have intense shaking chills—more than just shivering.

SEE YOUR DOCTOR TODAY:

- You're pregnant and have a fever.
- You have a fever of 101° F or higher and you're age 65 or older or have a chronic medical condition.
- You're coughing continuously. Or, you're coughing up colored sputum.

CALL YOUR DOCTOR OR NURSE HELP LINE:

- You're showing signs of the flu—or you've been exposed to the flu—and you have a weakened immune system, a chronic medical condition, live in a nursing home or are age 65 or older.
- You've had a fever for three or more days.
- You have flu symptoms that aren't getting better after several days.

TRY SELF-CARE:

- Try self-care only after you've seen or talked with your doctor.

SMART ACTIONS TODAY

If your symptoms indicate self-care:

Use OTC pain medications. They may help ease muscle, head and body aches. Follow the package directions carefully. Check with your doctor if you are pregnant or breast-feeding, or if you are not sure whether a certain medication is right for you. *Caution:* Never give aspirin to anyone younger than age 19. It's linked to a rare but sometimes fatal condition called Reye's syndrome.

Drink up. A fever may cause dehydration. So, drink enough water or other non-caffeinated liquids to stay hydrated.

Have a bowl of chicken soup. It restores salts and minerals that the virus may have depleted. This may help you feel better.

Take it easy. Bed rest allows your body to devote energy to healing. So, let your own natural defenses do their job. Also, you're still infectious for about five days after your symptoms appear. Be kind to others and stay home.

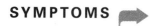

Practice flu etiquette. Cover your mouth and nose with a tissue when you cough or sneeze. Throw out the tissue immediately. Wash your hands as soon as possible. If tissues aren't handy, cough or sneeze into the upper part of your sleeve instead of directly into your hands.

MYTH OR TRUTH?

THE FLU SHOT WILL GIVE YOU THE FLU

MYTH. The flu shot does contain influenza viruses. But, these viruses have been killed and can no longer cause an infection. Approximately one in four people experiences soreness at the injection site. Some run a low-grade fever or feel achy for a day or two.

SMART ACTIONS TOMORROW

Ways to lessen your chance of coming down with the flu:

Get a second chance. If you're in a high-risk category and missed getting your vaccination early in the flu season, your doctor may consider prescribing one of several anti-viral oral medications that may protect you.

Clean often. Flu viruses may survive on surfaces for two to eight hours. Disinfect your home and your workplace often during flu season.

Take matters into your own hands. Touching a contaminated object, such as a doorknob or telephone, then touching your nose or mouth may spread the flu. The simple act of washing your hands reduces your risk of influenza significantly. Wash your hands with soap and warm water for 20 seconds. If water isn't available, use alcohol-based wipes or gel sanitizers.

Why the Flu Vaccine Is so Important

The single best way to avoid the flu is to get vaccinated every year. Once the vaccine is given, antibodies, or defenses, to the flu viruses develop within two weeks. There are two types of vaccines:

- The flu shot is an injection approved for use in healthy adults and adults with chronic medical conditions.
- The flu vaccine in nasal spray form is approved for use in healthy adults up to and including age 49. It should not be used by women who are pregnant, or by anyone with underlying medical conditions.

Who benefits?

Most people will benefit from getting vaccinated. In fact, the Centers for Disease Control and Prevention reports that the vaccine prevents the flu in an average of 80 percent of younger, healthy adults. However, talk with your doctor before getting the flu shot or nasal spray. Flu vaccinations may cause problems in some people. This is particularly true for those who've had a severe reaction to flu vaccinations in the past, those who are allergic to chicken eggs, or those with a history of Guillain-Barré syndrome.

Vaccination is especially important for:

- People who are at a high risk of flu complications or of catching or spreading the virus. This includes anyone who has a weakened immune system or an underlying health condition.
- Adults ages 50 and older
- Health care professionals
- Nursing home residents
- Pregnant women
- Anyone who lives with someone at high risk

Where to get vaccinated

Ask your doctor about giving you the flu vaccine. Or, to find a flu clinic near you, visit the American Lung Association's Web site at www.flucliniclocator.org.

INSECT BITES & STINGS

UNDERSTANDING YOUR SYMPTOMS

Insects may cause symptoms from a mild itch to a burning sting. Or, they may be more serious if you're allergic or if the insect carries a disease such as West Nile or Lyme. The most common biting and stinging bugs are mosquitoes, fleas, dust mites, honeybees and paper wasps. Bites and stings from yellow jackets, hornets, fire ants, ticks, and poisonous scorpions and spiders are also common.

Some poisonous spiders can be recognized by their markings. There are three in particular. The first is a black widow spider. It has a shiny black body and a red hourglass shape on its abdomen. The second, the brown recluse spider, is light brown, with skinny legs and a violin-shaped mark on its head. The last is the hobo spider, which is brown with chevron-shaped markings on its abdomen.

---

71 ▶ DECIDING YOUR NEXT STEP

CALL 911:

- You've had a severe allergic reaction to a sting in the past.
- You've been bitten or stung and have any of these signs of a life-threatening allergic reaction called anaphylaxis: a swollen throat or tongue; difficulty breathing or swallowing; stomach cramps; hives over a large area, or hives that are rapidly spreading; nausea or diarrhea; faintness, dizziness, chest pain or heart palpitations; you have a change in your level of consciousness.

SEEK EMERGENCY HELP:

- You're experiencing a high fever, headache, neck stiffness, tremors, muscle weakness or numbness. These are possible symptoms of the West Nile virus.
- You've been bitten by a poisonous spider or scorpion and are having muscle problems, excessive sweating, vision problems, fever, vomiting, new bruising or a severe headache.

SEE YOUR DOCTOR TODAY:

- You have several bee, wasp, hornet or yellow jacket stings.
- You have several fire-ant bites.
- You have a large amount of swelling at the sting site.
- You have a rapidly spreading area of skin that is red, swollen, hot and tender, or painful.
- You see red streaks or pus draining from the sting.
- You've been bitten or stung on your eyes, lips or genitalia, making it hard to see, eat or urinate.
- You have severe pain, despite treatment.

CALL YOUR DOCTOR OR NURSE HELP LINE:

- You have mild symptoms that last several days.
- You have a rash, muscle aches, swollen joints or flu-like symptoms.
- You've been bitten by a brown recluse or hobo spider. See Page 152 for tips on recognizing some types of spiders.

TRY SELF-CARE:

- You have pain but don't have any of the symptoms above.

Trend Line

Fewer than 5 percent of those stung by insects develop anaphylaxis. Source: American Academy of Allergy, Asthma & Immunology

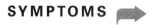
SMART ACTIONS NOW

If your symptoms indicate emergency care:

Get away. If the insect is still on you, stay calm as you brush it away. Then, move to a safer area.

Remove the stinger. Use your fingernail or a credit card to scrape out the stinger without squeezing more venom into your body. Speed is the key. Getting it out within 30 seconds helps prevent more venom from being released.

Give yourself an injection. If you've ever had a severe allergic reaction to an insect sting, you should have an up-to-date epinephrine kit with you at all times. Use it promptly after being stung. Then, seek emergency help.

If your symptoms indicate self-care:

Cool and elevate. Clean the area with mild soap and water. Then, apply a cool compress. Elevate the sting site. This will help lessen the amount of swelling and pain.

Stop the itch. Over-the-counter oral antihistamines, hydrocortisone cream or calamine lotion may help relieve itching. Follow the directions carefully. Ice, wrapped in a towel, also may help. Apply it to the affected area 10 to 15 minutes at a time, three to four times a day. Do this for the first 24 hours. If you have nerve damage, diabetes or poor circulation, check with your doctor first.

Remove ticks. Ticks can carry several diseases, including Lyme and Rocky Mountain spotted fever. Removing ticks as soon as possible may help prevent tick-borne diseases. So, it's important to remove them right away. Using tweezers, hold the tick as close to your skin as possible. Then, pull it straight out, removing its entire body. Next, wash the area with mild soap and water. If part of it remains under your skin, seek medical help to remove it.

SMART ACTIONS TOMORROW

It's hard to avoid all biting and stinging insects. But, here are some ways to protect yourself:

Keep your eyes open for nests. If you see any around your home, have them destroyed by a professional exterminator.

Shield yourself. Insect repellent will help you avoid bites from mosquitoes and ticks. It may be applied to your clothes and skin. Avoid your mouth and eyes. Wash your hands afterward. Experts recommend chemical products, such as DEET and Picaridin. They also recommend natural repellents such as oil of lemon eucalyptus. Be sure to read the label. Always follow the directions carefully.

Dress for protection. Long sleeves, pants, socks and closed-toe shoes may help prevent bites.

MYTH OR TRUTH?

WEST NILE—IF YOU HAVE IT, YOU KNOW IT

MYTH. Four out of five infected people have no symptoms. And, only 20 percent have mild symptoms, such as a fever, headache, body aches and nausea. About one in 150 infected people develops a severe illness. Source: Centers for Disease Control and Prevention

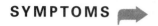

JOINT PAIN

UNDERSTANDING YOUR SYMPTOMS

If you have achy joints, there are a number of possible causes. Here are some of the more common ones:

- In osteoarthritis, wear and tear on a joint causes the cartilage to break down. This can result in a painful, stiff and sometimes tender or swollen joint.
- Gout is a type of arthritis. It's caused by a buildup of uric acid crystals in joints. It usually causes throbbing pain that occurs at night. Often, the pain is near the big toe. But, it may involve other joints.
- In rheumatoid arthritis (RA) and lupus, the body's immune system attacks its own healthy tissue. One of the results is joint pain. Other symptoms include fever and fatigue. Both conditions also may cause a low-grade fever.
- Septic arthritis starts when bacteria get into the joint.

Symptoms include pain, fever and joint swelling.

Other causes of joint pain may include viral infections, vaccinations, Lyme disease, trauma and overuse or sports injuries.

Trend Line

More than 21 percent of adults in the United States have some form of arthritis. It's estimated that the number of American adults with arthritis will increase by 40 percent by the year 2030. Source: American College of Rheumatology

72 ▶ DECIDING YOUR NEXT STEP

SEEK EMERGENCY HELP:

- You have severe pain when moving a joint that is red, swollen and warm.
- You have a fever of 104° F or higher.
- You have intense shaking chills—more than just shivering.

SEE YOUR DOCTOR TODAY:

- You have one or more joints that are red, swollen, warm, tender or painful.
- You have joint pain and a fever.
- You have new joint pain. You also have a compromised immune system, are an intravenous drug user, have a prosthetic, or have a joint that was already damaged by trauma or arthritis.

CALL YOUR DOCTOR OR NURSE HELP LINE:

- You have recently developed pain in more than one joint.
- You have pain that increases with joint movement.
- You have a bull's-eye rash, possibly around a recent tick bite.
- You have new joint pain and may have been bitten by a tick. Or, you've recently been in a tick-infested area.
- You have started a new medication.
- You have joint pain that has lasted for more than three days.

TRY SELF-CARE:

- You have mild joint pain but none of the symptoms above.

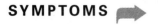
SMART ACTIONS TODAY

If your symptoms indicate self-care:

Use moist heat. If you know you have arthritis, try applying a heating pad with moisture to sore joints for 10 to 15 minutes at a time. Do this three or four times a day. Warm baths or showers may also help.

Seek pain relief. Over-the-counter pain relievers may help reduce stiffness, swelling and inflammation. Applying capsaicin cream to the sore joint may also help. Follow the package directions carefully. Check with your doctor if you are pregnant or breast-feeding, or if you're not sure whether a certain medication is safe for you. *Caution:* Never give aspirin to anyone younger than age 19. It's linked to a rare but sometimes fatal condition called Reye's syndrome.

SMART ACTIONS TOMORROW

If you have a chronic form of arthritis, talk with your doctor about trying to manage your condition through lifestyle changes. Try these tips:

Get enough shut-eye. During sleep, your body repairs itself. Rest may help you recover from an arthritis flare-up more quickly. It may even help prevent one. Aim for eight to 10 hours of sleep each night. Take naps as needed during the day.

Get moving. Regular exercise may help relieve joint stiffness, pain and fatigue. Low-impact aerobic activities, such as walking and swimming, are easier on sore joints. Talk with your doctor before starting any new exercise program. A physical therapist may help create an exercise program that's right for your needs.

Watch your weight. Extra pounds place added stress on joints. If you're overweight, losing weight may help reduce the pain. It also may keep osteoarthritis from getting worse.

Think about how you move. Avoid positions or movements that stress joints. Don't stand or sit in one position for a long period of time. To make everyday activities easier, consider home modifications. For example, installing grab bars in bathrooms may help.

Eat smart. Try to get enough calcium and vitamin D. For adults up to and including age 50, the recommended amount of calcium is 1,000 mg daily. For adults ages 51 and older it's 1,300 mg daily. The current recommended amounts of vitamin D for adults are between 400 and 800 international units (IU) daily. Pregnant women should ask their doctors about the right amount of calcium and vitamin D for them.

Ask about glucosamine. Glucosamine is naturally found in and around cartilage cells. Some experts believe the supplement form of glucosamine may help ease moderate to severe arthritis pain. But, not all experts agree. Ask your doctor if it's right for you.

MYTH OR TRUTH?

RHEUMATOID ARTHRITIS IS CRIPPLING
MYTH. Drug treatments have improved dramatically. Most newly diagnosed patients experience much less pain and swelling after starting treatment. They may then continue to go about their normal—or near normal—activity levels.

MALE GENITAL PROBLEMS

UNDERSTANDING YOUR SYMPTOMS

Genital symptoms may include pain and/or swelling in your scrotum, penis or genital area. You also may have a discharge from your penis. Or, you may have problems with erection or painful intercourse. Causes include: infections, ranging from jock itch to sexually transmitted diseases; genital injuries; hernias; and cancers of the prostate or testicles.

Testicular Pain?

If you're experiencing testicular pain, a medical evaluation is crucial. Don't delay. You may have a condition called testicular torsion, which can cut off blood to the testicles.

---

73 ▶ ## DECIDING YOUR NEXT STEP

SEEK EMERGENCY HELP:
- You have severe pain in your penis or groin.
- You have scrotal or testicular pain.
- You have sudden pain or swelling in your groin. It's accompanied by abdominal pain, nausea or vomiting.
- You have a hernia in your groin that does not go back into your abdomen when lying down. It's accompanied by abdominal pain, nausea or vomiting.
- Your scrotum or penis is black, blue or bright red.
- You have a prolonged, painful erection.
- You have something around your penis—such as a penile ring—that's causing swelling, or you're unable to remove.
- You have a fever of 104° F or higher.
- You have intense shaking chills—more than just shivering.

SEE YOUR DOCTOR TODAY:

- You have a penile discharge and a fever of 100.4° F or higher.
- You have an area that's red, swollen, hot and tender, or painful. Or, you see pus.
- You have a hernia in your groin that does not go back into your abdomen when lying down.

CALL YOUR DOCTOR OR NURSE HELP LINE:

- You find a lump in your scrotum. Or, your scrotum feels heavy.
- Your foreskin or the tip of your penis becomes swollen, red, sore or itchy.
- Your penis is swelling or you have a discharge. Or, you're unable to pull back the foreskin.
- You notice blood in your semen or a change in its color or amount.
- You find a genital lesion, sore or blister.
- You know or suspect you've been exposed to an STD.
- You have repeated difficulty having or maintaining an erection. Or, you have a painful erection.

TRY SELF-CARE:

- You have minor discomfort or other minor symptoms, or erectile trouble, but none of the symptoms above.

SMART ACTIONS TODAY

If your symptoms indicate self-care:

Rest. If you've been diagnosed with groin strain, rest and using an ice pack may help. Wrap the ice in a towel. Apply for 10 to 15 minutes. Repeat three to four times a day for the first 24 hours. If you have nerve damage, diabetes or poor circulation, check with your doctor first. Support your scrotum with an athletic supporter when moving around.

(Continued)

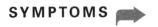

SMART ACTIONS TODAY *(Continued)*

Ease the pain. After your doctor has diagnosed your condition, over-the-counter (OTC) pain relievers may help. Follow the package directions carefully. Check with your doctor if you're not sure whether a certain medicine is safe for you. *Caution:* Never give aspirin to anyone younger than age 19. It's linked to a rare but sometimes fatal condition called Reye's syndrome.

Stay clean. For skin irritation, wash with mild soap, rinse and let air-dry. Avoid tight or damp clothes, scratching and public showers, pools and gyms.

Ditch the itch. Jock itch may be treated with an OTC antifungal cream, lotion, spray or powder that contains miconazole or clotrimazole. Follow the package directions.

SMART ACTIONS TOMORROW

Avoid some genital problems with these simple steps:

Protect yourself. If you're sexually active, you can help reduce your risk of STDs. Be sure to use a latex condom. If you're allergic to latex, use a polyurethane condom.

Get tested. If you've been exposed to an STD, avoid sexual activity until after you have been diagnosed and treated—and your condition has cleared. Your partner also should be evaluated and treated, as necessary.

Care for your foreskin. Clean an uncircumcised penis by sliding back the foreskin and washing with water only. And, pull back your foreskin when urinating.

Ask about self-exams. Experts disagree about the value of testicular self-examination (TSE). Ask your doctor if TSE is right for you.

MUSCLE PAIN

UNDERSTANDING YOUR SYMPTOMS

You've raked leaves or shoveled snow. Now your muscles are paying the price. Muscle pain may be caused by a simple strain. Or, your muscle pain may go along with pain in other connective tissue, such as ligaments and tendons. But, it also may be a sign of an infection or a chronic medical condition. It may even be a side effect of a medication. Some common causes:

- Autoimmune diseases, such as rheumatoid arthritis and polymyositis. These may inflame joints, tendons and muscles.
- Certain drugs. These may include cholesterol-lowering statins and illegal drugs.
- Fibromyalgia, a chronic disorder involving widespread pain and fatigue. Tender points may be in the neck, spine, shoulders and hips.
- Infections due to viruses, such as influenza. Or, it may be due to bacteria, such as those that cause Lyme disease.
- Injury or trauma, including bursitis, tendonitis, sprains and strains. See Sprains, Page 192.
- Overuse, from working a muscle too hard or too often.
- Repetitive motion disorders, such as carpal tunnel syndrome. These conditions are caused by longtime overuse of certain muscles.
- Tension or stress.

74 DECIDING YOUR NEXT STEP

SEEK EMERGENCY HELP:

- You're in severe pain.
- Your calf or thigh is painful, tender, red, warm or swollen—especially if you have a history of blood clots, or you are pregnant or have had any of the following in the last four weeks: trauma, chemotherapy, hospitalization, childbirth or surgery. Or, you have been immobilized or were sitting for a lengthy period, such as on a long flight.
- You have muscle pain along with new weakness.

SEE YOUR DOCTOR TODAY:

- You have muscle pain and an area that's red, swollen, hot, tender or painful.

CALL YOUR DOCTOR OR NURSE HELP LINE:

- You have frequent leg cramps.
- You have muscle cramps after starting a new medication.
- You have undiagnosed pain that lasts longer than 48 hours.
- You have persistent muscle pain and fever.
- You have unexplained, recurring muscle pain.
- Your pain is disrupting your daily life, including sleep.
- You have dark urine along with your muscle pain.
- You have a bull's eye rash, especially around a recent tick bite. Or, you've recently been in a tick-infested area.

TRY SELF CARE:

- You have occasional muscle cramps.
- Your muscle pain is the result of overuse.

SMART ACTIONS TODAY

If self-care is recommended:

Rest. Strained muscles need rest. Try to elevate the injured part above your heart to ease swelling. Over-the-counter (OTC) pain relievers may help. Follow the package directions carefully. Check with your doctor if you are pregnant or breast-feeding, or if you're not sure whether a certain medication is safe for you. *Caution:* Never give aspirin to anyone younger than age 19. It's linked to a rare but sometimes fatal condition called Reye's syndrome.

Ice. For the first 24 hours, use an ice pack. Wrap ice in a towel. Apply to sore muscles, 10 to 15 minutes at a time, three to four times a day. If you have nerve damage, diabetes or poor circulation, check with your doctor first. If you have an injured ankle, knee or wrist, mild compression with an elastic wrap, air cast or splint may help reduce swelling.

Stretch. If your pain is caused by cramps in the muscle, gentle stretching may help. For example, extend your leg and pull your foot back. Or, stand and press your foot against the floor to help relieve a leg cramp.

MYTH OR TRUTH?

NO PAIN, NO GAIN?

MYTH. Swinging right back into the activity that caused your pain could increase the chance of reinjury. Or, it may turn a onetime problem into a chronic issue. Give yourself time to rest and regain your range of motion, flexibility and strength. Gentle movement is fine. But, avoid high-impact aerobic activities, strenuous work or weight lifting while you're in pain.

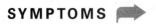

SMART ACTIONS TOMORROW

To help prevent muscle pain, adopt a healthful lifestyle and take a few precautions:

Stay active. Start or continue a regular exercise program. Strong, supple muscles are less prone to injury. Talk with your doctor before starting any new exercise program. Good choices are walking and swimming. When you exercise, always warm up. Be sure to drink enough fluids to stay hydrated. Avoid exercising or playing sports when you're tired or in pain.

Short-circuit cramps. Avoid sitting or standing in one position for too long. Take frequent stretching breaks when you're working. Also, do so if you're on a long car, bus or airplane trip. If you can't stand up, at least rotate your ankles and flex your calf muscles every hour to keep circulation flowing. Drink enough fluids to stay hydrated. That's because dehydration may cause muscles to cramp.

NASAL CONGESTION

UNDERSTANDING YOUR SYMPTOMS

It's hard to ignore a stuffed-up nose. Your nasal passages and sinuses may be congested due to a cold, allergies or sinusitis.

- If you have a cold, your symptoms may include a runny nose, scratchy throat and sneezing. Most colds are caused by a rhinovirus. These germs latch onto the cells that line your nose and sinuses. That causes lots of mucus discharge.

- If you have hay fever or other respiratory allergies—called allergic rhinitis—chances are you'll have the following symptoms: itchy, red, watery eyes; sneezing; a tickle in your throat; and a runny nose with clear, watery discharge. These symptoms are caused by sensitivity to allergens, such as pollen, dust, mold, dust mites, animal dander or even medications or foods. Sometimes allergy symptoms are hard to distinguish from a cold. The best clue: If your congestion always happens at the same time of year or always happens when you're exposed to the same substance, it's probably caused by allergies.

- If you have sinusitis, the mucous membranes in your nasal and sinus passages become inflamed and swollen. You may feel pressure around your eyes, nose, cheeks, upper jaw or even your teeth. You also may have a headache, watery eyes, yellowish green nasal discharge and a low-grade fever.

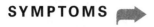

75 DECIDING YOUR NEXT STEP

SEEK EMERGENCY HELP:

- You have a fever of 104° F or higher.
- You have intense shaking chills—more than just shivering.
- You have a severe headache.
- You're having trouble seeing. Or, you can't move your eyes normally.
- You have a fever and neck pain or stiffness if you try to put your chin on your chest.
- If you're wheezing or having difficulty breathing, see Breathing Problems, Page 100.

SEE YOUR DOCTOR TODAY:

- You're pregnant and have a fever.
- You have a fever of 103° F or higher that doesn't respond to over-the-counter (OTC) medication.
- Your eyelids—or the area around your eyes—are swollen and painful.
- Your sinus pain is severe.
- You have a weakened immune system or diabetes.

CALL YOUR DOCTOR OR NURSE HELP LINE:

- You've had a fever for three days or longer.
- Your symptoms haven't improved—or have gotten worse—after several days.
- You're age 65 or older and have a fever.

TRY SELF-CARE:

- Your symptoms are mild.

SMART ACTIONS TODAY

If your symptoms indicate self-care:

Stay hydrated. Fluids help keep nasal secretions thin and loose. That makes it easier to break up congestion when you sneeze or blow your nose. Fluids also may soothe a scratchy throat. And, they lubricate mucous membranes.

Steam up. Breathing in warm, moist air may loosen mucus in your nasal and sinus passages. Stand in your bathroom while you run the shower. Or, fill a bowl with hot water. Then, cover your head with a towel. Lean over the bowl and breathe in deeply through your nose.

Ease the pain. OTC pain relievers and a warm compress may soothe sinus pain and headaches. Follow the package directions carefully. Check with your doctor if you are pregnant or breast-feeding, or if you're not sure whether a certain medication is safe for you. *Caution:* Never give aspirin to anyone younger than age 19. It's linked to a rare but sometimes fatal condition called Reye's syndrome.

Use decongestants wisely. A decongestant nasal spray may relieve swelling in your nasal passages. It also may help drainage. Don't use one for more than three days.

Be cautious with OTC cold remedies. Choose one that treats only the symptoms you have, with the least number of active ingredients. That will help minimize side effects and interactions with other medications you may be taking.

Consider an antihistamine for allergies. OTC antihistamines may lessen allergy symptoms. They come in liquids and tablets. Follow package directions carefully. Check labels for drowsiness warnings. Prescription nasal spray antihistamines may also help. Ask your doctor if they might be right for you.

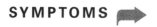

SMART ACTIONS TOMORROW

Steps to take to help minimize congestion:

Wash up. To kill germs, wash your hands frequently. Do so for 20 seconds each time with soap and warm water. If you're not near a sink, use alcohol-based disposable hand wipes or gel sanitizers.

Reduce your contact with allergens. Close your doors and windows during pollen season. If possible, install air conditioners and air filters to clean the air. Staying indoors as much as possible during the height of allergy season—and when the pollen count is high—helps, too.

Breathe easier while you sleep. If you're allergic to dust mites, enclosing your mattress and box springs in dust-proof materials may help. Washing your bed sheets every week in hot water may help, too.

Should You Take an Antibiotic?

Most likely, no. Colds and flu are spread by viruses, not bacteria. So, antibiotics will not help. In fact, taking them to treat a virus does more harm than good in the long run. That's because of the risk for building up an antibiotic resistance in the body. Every time you take an antibiotic, harmful bacteria are killed. But, some resistant germs may get left behind. These stubborn germs grow and multiply. The result could be that the next time you have a bacterial infection, the antibiotic won't be able to do its job.

NAUSEA & VOMITING

UNDERSTANDING YOUR SYMPTOMS

Nausea has many causes. Stomach disorders, food poisoning and motion sickness are a few. You may also have a virus that causes gastroenteritis. Some other causes include head injury, alcohol abuse, chemotherapy side effects or pancreatitis. Vomiting is often benign. But, it may have consequences, including dehydration and electrolyte abnormalities.

---

76 ▶ DECIDING YOUR NEXT STEP

CALL 911:
- You have nausea along with chest pain, pressure or discomfort. The pain may be in or move to your neck, jaw, throat, back, shoulders, abdomen or arms. Or, you're sweating and short of breath. You may be having a heart attack. See Chest Pain, Page 110.
- You have blood in your vomit. Or, the vomit looks like coffee grounds.
- You've fainted and you're vomiting.

SEEK EMERGENCY HELP:
- You're severely dehydrated, with extreme thirst or decreased urine output. You feel dizzy or faint when you stand.
- You have a fever of 104° F or higher.
- You have a head injury.
- You have diabetes and have labored breathing—and possibly fruity smelling breath—and are very ill.
- You're unable to keep down fluids for 12 hours or more.

(Continued)

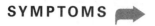

DECIDING YOUR NEXT STEP *(Continued)*

SEEK EMERGENCY HELP:
- You have severe or persistent abdominal pain.
- You're vomiting bile.

SEE YOUR DOCTOR TODAY:
- You're moderately dehydrated, with moderate thirst and infrequent urination. And, your urine may be dark yellow or amber.
- You have persistent nausea and a new headache.
- Your vomiting persists for a day or longer.

CALL YOUR DOCTOR OR NURSE HELP LINE:
- You've just started a new medication.
- Your nausea or vomiting makes you unable to take a prescribed medication.
- You have a weakened immune system or a chronic medical condition.
- Your nausea lasts three days or longer. Or, your nausea is a recurring problem.
- You're losing weight but don't know why.
- You have diabetes and have vomited more than once today.
- You're age 65 or older, are in ill health and have vomited more than once today.
- You're vomiting and have a fever of 101° F or higher for 48 hours or longer.
- You're vomiting and have a history of abdominal surgery.
- Your vomiting is self-induced.
- You tried self-care, but it didn't help.

TRY SELF-CARE:
- You have none of the symptoms above.
- You're mildly dehydrated, with slight thirst and slightly decreased urination.
- Your vomiting is due to motion sickness.

SMART ACTIONS TODAY

If your symptoms indicate self-care:

Get comfortable. Find the most comfortable position you can—sitting or lying down—in an area with fresh air and no strong odors. Take slow, deep breaths.

Stay hydrated. If you're vomiting, slowly sip small amounts of clear liquids. You also may suck on ice pops. Avoid diet sodas and beverages that have caffeine. Slowly, you may try larger sips of clear liquids.

Try ginger. This root may calm some types of nausea. Ask your doctor if ginger products are a good option for you. Ginger products may be found in health food stores.

Keep it bland. If you've been free of vomiting for six hours, slowly start to eat some bland foods. Bananas, applesauce, rice, soda crackers or toast are good choices. Avoid high-fat foods.

Banish germs. Wash your hands often with soap and warm water for 20 seconds. Disinfect surfaces, such as door handles and countertops.

SMART ACTIONS TOMORROW

Steps to keep nausea to a minimum:

Avoid motion sickness. Eat a light snack before traveling. Skip spicy, greasy or acidic foods. In a car, the front seat is best. If you're not driving, close your eyes or scan the horizon. Open the window and recline. On a plane, try to sit above the wing. On a boat, choose the front or middle.

Keep a diary. It may help identify the cause of the vomiting. List what you've eaten, and any medications you've taken.

NOSEBLEEDS

UNDERSTANDING YOUR SYMPTOMS

Our noses are lined with tiny blood vessels. Even minor trauma to those blood vessels, such as several sneezes in a row, may cause bleeding. Here are some other common causes of nosebleeds:

- A deviated septum may cause blockages that make sinus infections and nosebleeds more common.
- Irritated nasal tissues may result in crusts forming inside your nose. Many things can cause irritation, including allergies, a cold or a sinus infection. Others are nasal sprays—including intranasal steroids—or dry heat and low humidity in the winter. When you sneeze, blow or rub your nose, these crusts may bleed. Smoking and secondhand smoke also may irritate nasal passages, making you more susceptible to nosebleeds.
- Minor or serious nose injuries may cause a nosebleed. These can range from a broken nose to nasal surgery. Forcefully blowing or picking your nose is another cause.
- Problems with blood clotting also may cause nosebleeds.

Trend Line

About 60 percent of Americans have regular nosebleeds, and for the vast majority, nosebleeds are nothing to worry about. Source: American Academy of Family Physicians

DECIDING YOUR NEXT STEP

SEEK EMERGENCY HELP:

- You have uncontrolled nose bleeding despite applying pressure.
- Your nose is bleeding as the result of an accident, fall or head injury.
- The nosebleed began with blood draining down your throat, not out of your nostrils.

SEE YOUR DOCTOR TODAY:

- Your nosebleed doesn't stop after two 10-minute pinching sessions.
- You're vomiting blood as a result of your nosebleed.
- Your nosebleed recurs more than twice in a 24-hour period, despite treatment.
- You have a bleeding disorder. Or, you take a blood thinner such as aspirin or warfarin (Coumadin).

CALL YOUR DOCTOR OR NURSE HELP LINE:

- You have frequent nosebleeds for no apparent reason.
- You have high blood pressure, liver disease or kidney disease, or have had recent chemotherapy.
- You use a steroid nasal spray and have frequent nosebleeds.
- You are age 65 or older.
- In addition to nosebleeds, you have easy bruising. Or, you frequently have bleeding gums.

TRY SELF-CARE:

- You have none of the above symptoms and your nose stops bleeding when you pinch it for 10 to 20 minutes.

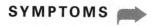

SMART ACTIONS TODAY

If your symptoms indicate self-care:

Stop it with a pinch. Squeeze your nostrils shut using your thumb and finger. Sit up straight and lean your head forward. Breathe through your mouth. Don't lie down or tilt your head back. Swallowing blood may cause nausea or vomiting. Apply continuous pressure for 10 minutes. Then, check to see if the bleeding has stopped. If it hasn't, very gently blow your nose to remove clots. Then, pinch your nostrils shut again for another 10 minutes.

Leave it alone. Don't place gauze, ice or other objects inside your nose. Once bleeding has stopped, don't sniff or blow your nose for several hours. If you must sneeze, keep your mouth open. That will put less pressure on your nose.

Take it easy. For two to three days after a nosebleed, avoid strenuous exercise, lifting heavy objects, bending over and straining.

MYTH OR TRUTH?

NOSEBLEEDS ARE KID STUFF
MYTH. Though nosebleeds are more common in children younger than age 10, anyone can have one. And, the incidence of nosebleeds peaks in adults again after they reach age 50.

SMART ACTIONS TOMORROW

Help prevent nosebleeds with a few simple measures:

Moisture helps. Heated air in the winter and dry climates may dry out your nose. Use a humidifier to help moisten the air. Clean it daily or as instructed by the manufacturer. In winter, try dabbing petroleum jelly at the opening of your nostrils twice a day. Or, use a spritz of over-the-counter (OTC) saline nasal spray or mist—*not* a decongestant spray—two or three times a day. This may be especially helpful when traveling on airplanes, where air tends to be dry.

Consider your nasal spray. OTC decongestant sprays and some prescription nasal sprays may injure your nose. They also increase the chance of a nosebleed.

Protect your nose. Wear a helmet or face mask when playing sports that could result in an injury to your face. This may include baseball, football or hockey.

Stay infection-free. To help prevent colds and sinus infections that may result in nosebleeds, wash your hands frequently. Use soap and warm water for 20 seconds. A hand sanitizer is a good option when you're not near a sink. Get eight hours or more of sleep each night. And, ask your doctor if you should get a flu or pneumonia vaccine.

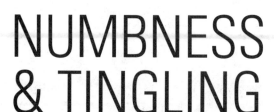

NUMBNESS & TINGLING

UNDERSTANDING YOUR SYMPTOMS

There are many possible causes for numbness and tingling. Here are some of the more common ones:

- You stayed still, in the same position, for too long. Numbness and tingling may simply be a sign that you've temporarily placed pressure on one of your nerves. Move around to increase circulation.

- Repetitive stress—such as from typing, operating a jackhammer, sewing, painting, working on an assembly line, or doing any motion over and over again—may cause swelling, weakness, numbness and tingling in your hands and fingers. Carpal tunnel syndrome occurs when the nerve that passes through your wrist and gives sensation to your fingers becomes compressed from swelling. This makes your hand, wrist and arm feel numb and painful.

- A herniated disk may cause numbness, tingling and pain. This happens when the disks between the bones of your spine protrude and squeeze the nerves. When a disk protrudes in your lower back, pain may radiate down your buttocks, legs and feet. When a disk protrudes in your neck, you may feel pain in your shoulders, neck or arms. You also may feel numbness and tingling down one arm.

- An injured nerve from a neck injury may cause numbness and tingling along your arms or hands. A low back injury may cause numbness and tingling down your legs.

- Damage to the peripheral nervous system (nerves from the brain or spinal cord) can result in numbness, tingling or pain. This damage or injury to the nerves is called peripheral neuropathy.

- In spinal stenosis, pressure is placed on the nerve roots and spinal cord due to spinal narrowing. This can lead to numbness, pain and weakness. It's most common in people ages 50 and older.

78 DECIDING YOUR NEXT STEP
CALL 911:
- You're experiencing a sudden onset of the following symptoms, which may indicate a stroke: numbness or weakness, especially in your face, arms or legs; trouble with your balance or coordination; difficulty with speaking or understanding other people's speech; confusion; trouble seeing in one or both eyes.

SEEK EMERGENCY HELP:
- Your arms or legs suddenly turn pale, blue or gray. This may indicate impaired circulation.

SEE YOUR DOCTOR TODAY:
- You have numbness or tingling that's not related to sitting or sleeping in one position.

CALL YOUR DOCTOR OR NURSE HELP LINE:
- Your numbness or tingling occurred after using a prescription medication.
- Your fingers turn pale and tingle when exposed to the cold.
- You have recurring episodes of numbness or tingling.

TRY SELF-CARE
- You don't have any of the symptoms described above.

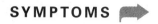
SMART ACTIONS TODAY

If your symptoms indicate self-care:

Get going. Does an arm or leg feel numb after you've been sitting for a while or sleeping? Change your position or get up and walk around.

Ease swelling. If your hands are feeling swollen, numb and painful from doing the same activity over and over again, an over-the-counter pain reliever may help. Follow the package directions carefully. Check with your doctor if you are pregnant or breast-feeding, or if you're not sure whether a certain medication is safe for you. *Caution:* Never give aspirin to anyone younger than age 19. It's linked to a rare but sometimes fatal condition called Reye's syndrome.

MYTH OR TRUTH?

COMPUTER TIME = CARPAL TUNNEL

MYTH. People who work on an assembly line are three times more likely to develop carpal tunnel syndrome than data-entry workers.

Source: National Institute of Neurological Disorders and Stroke

SMART ACTIONS TOMORROW

Try these steps to help reduce the frequency and severity of numbness and tingling:

Check your workstation. To reduce stress on your wrists, make sure your workstation is ergonomically correct. At the computer, place the keyboard low enough that your wrists are straight when you type. Use a mouse pad with a cushion that supports your wrist.

Consider a splint. This may take pressure away from your nerves and muscles. If you've been diagnosed with carpal tunnel syndrome, a splint may also relieve pain and numbness. As often as possible, try to rest the area that hurts by taking frequent breaks.

Rest. If repetitive movements are causing numbness and tingling, try to take frequent breaks to rest your hands.

Power up. If you work repeatedly with hand tools such as screwdrivers, use power tools, if possible. This will cut down on the number of times you have to twist your wrist. And, when you're buying any kind of hand tool, look for one that fits well in your hand.

RAPID HEARTBEAT

UNDERSTANDING YOUR SYMPTOMS

Your heart normally beats 60 to 100 times a minute. That's about 100,000 times a day. Most of the time you barely notice it. But, there are also times when you may feel your heart pounding in your chest. Or, you may hear it thumping in your ears. Fortunately, most causes of rapid, or irregular, heartbeat are not due to disease. They may include exercise, use of caffeine or tobacco, over-the-counter medications, and anxiety or stress. Certain prescription drugs, diet pills and over-the-counter supplements also may increase heart rate.

Health problems such as fever and overactive thyroid (hyperthyroidism) also may cause your heart to beat faster or irregularly. So may other conditions, such as coronary artery disease, heart attack and even heart failure.

---

79 ▶ ## DECIDING YOUR NEXT STEP
CALL 911:

- You have a rapid heartbeat and shortness of breath, chest pain or pressure, excessive sweating, fatigue, dizziness or lightheadedness.
- You have signs of shock. This may include a rapid heartbeat, rapid breathing, low blood pressure, faintness, confusion, lack of alertness, sweating, pale skin and a weak pulse.
- You have an implanted defibrillator or pacemaker and are receiving frequent shocks. Or, you have recurrent or persistent episodes of rapid heartbeat.

- You have signs of heart failure, including a racing heart, shortness of breath, difficulty breathing when you lie down, and heart palpitations. Other signs: You're coughing up a frothy, blood-tinged mucus. You've gained weight from retaining fluid. You've stopped urinating as much as normal. Or, you're fatigued, weak and feeling faint.

SEEK EMERGENCY HELP:
- You have a rapid heartbeat and a history of heart problems, a family history of sudden death, or you are frail.

SEE YOUR DOCTOR TODAY:
- You have a new, persistent occurrence of rapid heart rate. Or, your heartbeat is irregular.
- You're pregnant and have a new onset of rapid heart rate.
- You have an implanted pacemaker and have an irregular heartbeat or your heart rate changes from its usual range.

CALL YOUR DOCTOR OR NURSE HELP LINE:
- You frequently notice your heart skipping beats or frequently speeding up without an obvious cause, such as exercise or anxiety.
- You have symptoms of an overactive thyroid. These may include a rapid heartbeat, weight loss, sweating, nervousness, hand tremors and trouble sleeping.
- You've started a new medication.

TRY SELF-CARE:
- Because serious health problems are often caused by a rapid or irregular heartbeat, don't try to treat this condition without medical help.

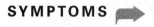

MYTH OR TRUTH?

FUMES MAY AFFECT HEART RATE

TRUTH. Things you inhale—such as car emissions, cigarette smoke, pollution, paint thinner and propane-gas fumes—may all cause your heart to beat faster.

SMART ACTIONS TOMORROW

To help lower your chances of having a racing heart:

Live healthfully. A low-fat diet may help prevent heart disease and other heart problems, including a rapid or irregular heartbeat. Lots of fruits and vegetables are good, too. Lose extra weight and keep it off. And, don't smoke.

Limit caffeine and alcohol. Talk with you doctor about what amounts—if any—are OK for you. Remember: Many foods and beverages contain caffeine. These include chocolate and many teas and soft drinks.

Get moving. People who exercise have lower resting heart rates. Aim for at least 30 minutes of aerobic exercise on most days of the week. Walking and swimming are good choices. Do resistance training, or weight lifting, two or three days a week. Talk with your doctor before starting any new exercise program. This is especially important if you've had a rapid heartbeat.

Quick Tip

It's normal for your heart to beat faster during exercise. Make sure it doesn't go too high by learning your target heart rate. To learn how to find your target zone, see Page 27. If you're over your target, try lowering the intensity of your workout.

RASHES

UNDERSTANDING YOUR SYMPTOMS

Rashes are quite common and can have a variety of causes. They may be itchy, burning or stinging. Here's a look at some, but not all, causes:

- Eczema is an inflammation of the skin. There are many different types of eczema. One common type is atopic dermatitis. It causes an itchy, red rash. Sometimes it's found in the folds of your arms, behind your knees or on your hands and scalp. Contact dermatitis causes itchy bumps or blisters, and dry patches. Skin color changes also may appear in areas where your skin is exposed to an allergen. These include detergents, cosmetics, metals and other materials.

- Touching poison ivy, sumac or oak plants may cause a rash. These plants have an oil that most people react to within a day or two of touching it. Redness and swelling are the first signs. A day later, small, itchy blisters may appear. These will last for about a week.

- Some illnesses, insect bites or medications may cause itchy red blotches called hives.

- A latex allergy may cause a rash and asthma when you touch this material. It's often found in gloves, condoms, balloons, rubber bands, shoe soles and more.

- Hot tub dermatitis may make your skin itchy with a bumpy red rash. When hot tubs and spas are poorly maintained, irritating germs may grow in the water.

- Other rashes can be due to autoimmune disorders, acne and infectious diseases.

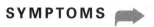
80 ▶ DECIDING YOUR NEXT STEP

CALL 911:

- You have hives and any of these signs of a life-threatening allergic reaction called anaphylaxis: a swollen throat or tongue; difficulty breathing or swallowing; stomach cramps; nausea or diarrhea; faintness, dizziness, chest pain or heart palpitations; you have a change in your level of consciousness.
- You're extremely ill. And, you develop widespread bruising or a purplish, pinpoint rash that doesn't lose its color when pressed. This may indicate bleeding under the skin due to a clotting problem or body-wide infection.

SEEK EMERGENCY HELP:

- You have a fever of 104° F or higher.

SEE YOUR DOCTOR TODAY:

- You've been exposed to poison ivy. And, you have a rash over a large part of your body.
- You have a rash near your eyes, mouth or genitals.
- You have a rapidly spreading rash that is red, swollen, hot and tender, or painful, or red streaks develop.
- Your rash is leaking pus from its blisters. Or, you have widespread fluid-filled blisters.
- You have a bright red rash that peels off in sheets.
- You have a fever of 102° F or higher. Or, have a fever and are: age 65 or older, pregnant, or have a weakened immune system.
- You have signs of shingles: a stinging, burning rash that begins as red bumps and turns into blisters after a few days. This usually occurs in people ages 50 and older who have had chicken pox.

CALL YOUR DOCTOR OR NURSE HELP LINE:

- You have hives that keep coming back.

- You're pregnant, age 65 or older, or have a weakened immune system.
- You've started a new medication.
- You have a rash, one that's painful or an itchy rash that doesn't respond to self-care. Or, you develop a bull's-eye rash, especially around the site of a recent tick bite.

TRY SELF-CARE:
- You have mild itching or skin redness but none of the above symptoms.

SMART ACTIONS TODAY

If your symptoms indicate self-care:

Stop scratching. Scratching at any type of rash may break the skin. This may lead to an infection.

Ease the itch. Hydrocortisone creams, calamine lotion and oatmeal baths may help. For eczema, try a moisturizer to help prevent itching. But, only use these products if you don't have broken skin. Also, keep cool. Warm temperatures and sweating may irritate a rash.

Halt hives. Oral—not topical—antihistamines may help relieve itchy hives. Follow package directions carefully. Check with your doctor if you're pregnant or breast-feeding, or if you're not sure whether a certain medication is safe for you.

MYTH OR TRUTH?

HOT TUBS MAY CAUSE RASHES
TRUTH. If you have a hot tub, test the chlorine or bromine levels and the water pH frequently. Warmer water causes chlorine and disinfectants to break down more quickly. That leaves you exposed to germs that may cause a rash.

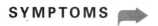

SMART ACTIONS TOMORROW

Take these steps to help prevent rashes and skin irritation:

Watch what you touch. Avoid things that irritate your skin. This includes cleaning solutions, gasoline and turpentine. Or, wear protective gloves when working with or around these types of things. If you have eczema, stop working and remove your gloves now and then. This is so your hands won't perspire, since moisture may worsen eczema. If you're allergic to latex, avoid products that contain it, such as certain sterile gloves, condoms, balloons and rubber bands. Also, be sure to tell your doctor, dentist and other health care professionals if you have a latex allergy.

Shower smart. Shower in cool or warm—not hot—water. Use a mild soap or a soap substitute. When drying off, pat skin dry—don't rub. Follow immediately with unscented lotion to seal in moisture. Or, take an occasional bath. Soaking in warm water for a short period of time helps skin absorb more moisture.

Keep skin moist. Dry skin may make eczema worse. A plain moisturizer may help. Try petroleum jelly or another fragrance-free, alcohol-free moisturizer. In winter, use a cool-mist humidifier to keep indoor air moist. Be sure to clean and maintain it according to the manufacturer's directions. Wear gloves when outside.

Know your poison. In the United States, poison ivy either grows low to the ground or winds up trees. It has three leaves on every stem. Don't touch it with your skin, clothes or shoes. And, don't touch anything else that may have come in contact with it.

SORE THROAT

UNDERSTANDING YOUR SYMPTOMS

A sore throat is not only uncomfortable, it also makes it painful to swallow. Depending on the cause, your sore throat may feel worse in the morning and improve as the day progresses. It usually results from inflammation of a part of the throat called the pharynx.

Most sore throats are caused by viruses. But, they're also caused by bacteria, most commonly strep. Other possible causes include allergies, post nasal drip, mononucleosis and heartburn. Sore throats may have environmental causes, too. These include tobacco smoke, smog, dust or excessively dry air. A sore throat may even result from a recent surgery, such as a tonsillectomy or adenoidectomy.

---

81 ▶ DECIDING YOUR NEXT STEP

CALL 911:
- You're completely unable to swallow and may also be drooling due to throat swelling.
- You're very ill and have a purplish, pinpoint rash that doesn't lose color if you press on it. You also may have unusual bruising.
- If you're wheezing or having difficulty breathing, see Breathing Problems, Page 100.

SEEK EMERGENCY HELP:
- You have a fever of 104° F or higher.
- You have a fever and severe neck pain or stiffness when you try to place your chin on your chest.
- You have difficulty or pain opening your mouth. And, your voice may be muffled due to throat swelling.

(Continued)

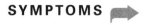

DECIDING YOUR NEXT STEP *(Continued)*

SEE YOUR DOCTOR TODAY:

- You've had a fever of 103° F or higher and fever reducers haven't worked.
- You're pregnant and have a fever in addition to a sore throat.
- You have a severe sore throat that is not responding to self-care.
- You have diabetes or a weakened immune system.

CALL YOUR DOCTOR OR NURSE HELP LINE:

- You've had a fever of 101° F or higher for 24 hours or longer.
- You have a sore throat with any other symptoms. These may include sandpaper rash on your chest or abdomen; stomachache; vomiting; tender or swollen glands; or white spots in the back of your throat.
- You've had a sore throat for at least three days. Or, you've been on an antibiotic for two days without any improvement.
- You have a history of rheumatic fever and you aren't on a preventive antibiotic therapy.

TRY SELF-CARE:

- You have none of the symptoms above.

MYTH OR TRUTH?

STOP ANTIBIOTICS ONCE YOUR THROAT FEELS BETTER

MYTH. If you are diagnosed with strep throat and are taking prescribed antibiotics, it's extremely important to finish the entire prescription, even if you feel better before all of the medicine runs out.

SMART ACTIONS TODAY

If your symptoms indicate self-care:

Rest and stay hydrated. Get plenty of rest. Eat a soft diet for one or two days. Drink enough fluids to stay hydrated, especially if you also have a fever. Try clear fruit juice, herbal tea, or hot water with lemon juice and honey. Ice pops or ice chips may also help. Skip acidic beverages such as orange juice, as well as spicy foods.

Try using a cool mist humidifier. This may help keep your mucous membranes moist and less irritated, especially if you tend to breathe through your mouth. Clean and maintain the humidifier according to the manufacturer's directions.

Consider a saline gargle. It may comfort a sore throat. Mix one-half teaspoon of salt in 8 ounces of warm water and gargle with it three or four times a day. Also, don't smoke. And, avoid smoke-filled rooms.

Ease the pain. Over-the-counter pain relievers may help ease your discomfort. Follow the package directions carefully. Check with your doctor if you are pregnant or breast-feeding, or if you're not sure whether a certain medication is safe for you. *Caution:* Never give aspirin to anyone younger than age 19. It's linked to a rare but sometimes fatal condition called Reye's syndrome.

SMART ACTIONS TOMORROW

Use this tip to reduce your risk of a sore throat:

Wash your hands often. This is one of the best things you can do to prevent the spread of germs. Wash your hands before eating, after using the bathroom and during cold-and-flu season. Use soap and warm water for 20 seconds. Dry hands thoroughly.

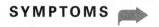

SPRAINS

UNDERSTANDING YOUR SYMPTOMS

Ligaments are tough tissues that hold your bones together at the joints. You probably don't think much about them until you experience a sprain. If you fall, or suddenly twist a joint, you may stretch or tear the ligaments that keep the joint in place. When a sprain happens, you may feel a pop, tear or pain. Swelling and bruising will follow. You may have trouble moving the joint or putting weight on it. Your joint also may feel loose or weak.

Sprains to the ankle, knee, wrist and thumb are often due to a fall or sports injury. Low back sprains may happen if you lift something the wrong way. The neck may become sprained due to a car accident or hard fall.

MYTH OR TRUTH?

A STRAIN IS A SPRAIN

MYTH. Although some of the symptoms are similar, a strain is different from a sprain. A strain occurs when a muscle or tendon is stretched, twisted or torn. A sprain, on the other hand, affects a ligament. Strains may cause pain, swelling, cramping, reduced movement, muscle spasms and weakness.

82 **DECIDING YOUR NEXT STEP**

SEEK EMERGENCY HELP:
- You have a severe sprain and can't put weight on the joint.
- You have sudden paralysis or loss of feeling in the injured joint.
- You're in severe pain.
- Your joint is bent in an odd way. Or, you suspect you have broken a bone. See Bone Injuries—Extremities, Page 98.

SEE YOUR DOCTOR TODAY:
- You have immediate, extensive rapid swelling or bruising.
- Your pain isn't relieved by treatment.
- Your injury occurred along with a popping sound or snapping sensation.

CALL YOUR DOCTOR OR NURSE HELP LINE:
- The part of your body that's injured has already been injured several times.
- You have no improvement 72 hours after your injury.

TRY SELF-CARE:
- You have a mild sprain that responds well to self-care. And, you aren't experiencing any of the symptoms above.

Trend Line

On any given day in the United States, more than 25,000 people sprain an ankle. Source: National Institutes of Health

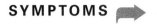

SMART ACTIONS TODAY

If your symptoms indicate self-care:

Try RICE. During the first 24 to 48 hours after a sprain, follow the RICE formula — rest, ice, compress, elevate. This will help reduce swelling and pain. Avoid placing weight on the affected joint. And, limit joint activity. Apply an ice pack — wrapped in a towel — or cold compress. Do this for 10 to 15 minutes, three to four times a day for the first 24 hours. If you have nerve damage, diabetes or poor circulation, check with your doctor first. Keep the injured joint wrapped in a bandage or splint. Keep it elevated above your heart when possible.

Stop the pain. Taking an over-the-counter pain reliever may help relieve pain and swelling. Follow the package directions carefully. Check with your doctor if you are pregnant or breast-feeding, or if you're not sure whether a certain medication is safe for you. *Caution:* Never give aspirin to anyone younger than age 19. It's linked to a rare but sometimes fatal condition called Reye's syndrome.

Ease back into action. After 48 hours, your doctor may recommend exercises that will help your joint become flexible and strong again. Or, he or she may recommend physical therapy. Your doctor or physical therapist will let you know when you may go back to your normal activities, including playing sports. This is usually three to six weeks after a mild sprain and up to a year later for a severe one.

SMART ACTIONS TOMORROW

Take these precautions to prevent a sprain:

Exercise smart. With your doctor's OK, regular exercise strengthens your muscles and keeps you in good shape. But, listen to your body. Working out when you're tired or in pain makes you more likely to sprain something. Always warm up before workouts. For five to 10 minutes, walk or do other light activity. If you've had sprains in the past, ask your doctor what exercises are best for you. Also, ask whether you should use a brace or athletic tape to prevent reinjury.

Prevent back sprains. Doing crunches or other exercises that strengthen your abdominal muscles will help your spine remain strong and stable. Talk with your doctor before starting any new exercise program. This is especially important if you have osteoporosis or another back condition. Losing weight also may help take the strain off your lower back. For more healthy back tips, see Back Pain—Low, Page 94.

Walk carefully. Only wear shoes that offer good support. Make sure all shoes fit comfortably. Check that the heels haven't worn down on one side. Whenever possible, avoid walking on uneven surfaces.

Prevent slips. Wipe up spills on the floor right away. In winter, use sand or rock salt to melt ice on your walkways. Use nonskid pads to keep rugs in place. And, keep stairs, walkways and driveways free of clutter.

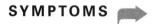

SUNBURNS

UNDERSTANDING YOUR SYMPTOMS

Everyone, regardless of skin color, can get a sunburn. However, some people are more vulnerable than others. For example, sun exposure history or certain complexions can increase risk. Typically, the telltale signs of a sunburn are redness and tenderness. But, a severe sunburn also may cause blisters, nausea, fever and chills. As soon as you notice any symptoms, take action quickly to prevent further skin damage and help ease your discomfort.

Sunburned skin may peel off in a few days, revealing a new layer of tender skin. But, that doesn't erase the damage. The sun's ultraviolet (UV) rays may permanently damage the underlying tissue. The most serious consequence of sunburn is that you increase your risk of developing skin cancer. Another negative effect is that sunburn prematurely ages your skin, making it look leathery, wrinkled and spotted.

---

83 ► ## DECIDING YOUR NEXT STEP
SEEK EMERGENCY HELP:
- Blisters from your sunburn cover a large area of skin.
- You have a fever of 101° F or higher.
- You're feeling faint, dizzy or nauseated.

SEE YOUR DOCTOR TODAY:
- Your pain lasts for two or more hours despite taking pain medication.
- You have blisters on your face or ears.
- You have increasing swelling, redness or drainage.

CALL YOUR DOCTOR OR NURSE HELP LINE:

- You have a weakened immune system or a chronic medical condition, such as diabetes.
- Your pain has lasted for more than 48 hours.
- The sunburn hasn't healed after one week.
- You have a large number of blisters.
- You haven't had a tetanus shot within the past five years, you haven't completed the tetanus series, you're not sure when you had your last tetanus shot, or you have a weakened immune system.

TRY SELF-CARE:

- Your skin is red, mildly swollen and tender without extreme pain. Or, you just have a few blisters.

SMART ACTIONS TODAY

If your symptoms indicate self-care:

Keep cool. Take a cool bath without soap. For additional relief, you may add 1 cup of baking soda or an oatmeal bath product to the water. Cool compresses also may ease the pain. Try a bath or compresses for 10 to 15 minutes, several times a day. Then, moisturize with aloe vera gel or lotion.

Ease the pain. An over-the-counter pain medication may relieve the discomfort. Follow the package directions carefully. Check with your doctor if you are pregnant or breast-feeding, or if you're not sure whether a certain medication is safe for you. *Caution:* Never give aspirin to anyone younger than age 19. It's linked to a rare but sometimes fatal condition called Reye's syndrome.

Leave blisters alone. Never break blisters. If they break accidentally, gently wash the area. Apply a topical antibiotic ointment. Then, cover with a clean bandage.

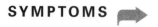
SMART ACTIONS TOMORROW

Sound advice to help you enjoy the sun:

Apply sun protection. Use sunscreen labeled *broad spectrum.* That means it protects against both UVA and UVB rays. Look for a sun protection factor (SPF) rating of 30 or higher. Reapply as directed. Lip balm with sunscreen should be used, too.

Check your meds. Some medications and cosmetics may make your skin more sensitive to UV rays. Check the labels for indications, or ask your pharmacist or doctor.

Watch the clock. Avoid or limit your time in the sun between 10 a.m. and 4 p.m. This is when the rays are most intense.

Dress for protection. When it's practical, wear clothing that helps block more of the sun's rays. Long-sleeved shirts or pants are best. Dry, dark and tightly woven fabrics offer the most UV protection. Hats with 2- to 3-inch brims protect your face, eyes, neck and ears.

Wear sunglasses. The most effective sunglasses offer 98 to 100 percent protection from UVA and UVB radiation.

MYTH OR TRUTH?

TANNING BEDS ARE SAFER THAN THE SUN

MYTH. Tanning beds, booths and lamps produce the same harmful ultraviolet radiation as the sun. In fact, indoor tanning may expose your skin to even stronger radiation than the sun.

URINARY PROBLEMS

UNDERSTANDING YOUR SYMPTOMS

There are many types and causes of urinary problems.

- A urinary tract infection may create an urge to urinate. It also may cause pain or burning when urinating. Back pain and cloudy or even blood-tinged urine are other possible signs. Bacteria are usually the cause. Most infections start in the urethra. But, they also may involve the bladder and kidneys. Left untreated, such infections may lead to kidney damage.

- A frequent urge to urinate may be the result of drinking too much caffeine or alcohol, being pregnant or taking diuretic drugs. But, it also may be a symptom of undiagnosed or uncontrolled diabetes. Or, it may be a sign of a kidney problem or other medical problem.

- Difficulty with bladder control during pregnancy, childbirth and menopause may affect some women. In some men, bladder leaks may be a result of an enlarged prostate. Bladder trouble also may be a side effect of prostate cancer treatments.

---

84 ⮞ ## DECIDING YOUR NEXT STEP
SEEK EMERGENCY HELP:

- You have intense shaking chills—more than just shivering.
- You can't release any urine from your bladder.
- You have extreme weakness and difficulty functioning.
- You have severe abdominal pain. Or, pain that's worse when you move.

(Continued)

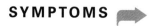
DECIDING YOUR NEXT STEP *(Continued)*

SEE YOUR DOCTOR TODAY:

- You're pregnant.
- You're nauseous or vomiting.
- You have severe pain when you urinate. Or, you have abdominal, low back or groin pain.
- You have a fever of 101° F or higher.
- Your urine is pink, red or brown. And, you take a blood thinner or have a bleeding disorder.
- You have a weakened immune system.
- Your urinary problems started after a recent gynecologic or urologic procedure or surgery.

CALL YOUR DOCTOR OR NURSE HELP LINE:

- Your urine is light pink, red, dark or cloudy. Or, it smells very bad.
- There has been a change in the frequency, urgency or amount of your urine.
- You have pain or burning when you urinate.
- You've been treated for a urinary tract infection (UTI). But, you aren't improving after 24 to 48 hours.
- There is unusual drainage or discharge from your vagina or penis.
- You leak urine when you laugh, walk or lift a heavy object. Or, you leak when your bladder is full.

TRY SELF-CARE:

- You've talked with your doctor about your symptoms. He or she has recommended self-care.

SMART ACTIONS TODAY

If your symptoms indicate self-care:

Drink enough fluids. Extra liquid may flush bacteria out of your bladder when you have an infection. Drink water and fruit juices. Avoid caffeine and alcohol. They may irritate your bladder.

Urinate when the urge strikes. Bacteria may grow in urine that's left in your bladder too long. So, go when you feel the urge. Don't hold it in.

Try a sitz bath. Soak in only a few inches of warm water. This may help ease UTI pain. If you're pregnant, check with your doctor first.

MYTH OR TRUTH?

CRANBERRY JUICE HELPS PREVENT UTIs

TRUTH. Compounds in cranberries make the bladder wall slippery. So, bacteria can't latch on. Choose real cranberry juice or cranberry capsules. Don't choose sweetened cocktails. But, before using cranberry juice or capsules for UTI prevention, check with your doctor. This is key if you take prescription medicines, have diabetes, have had kidney stones or have any dietary restrictions.

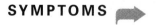

SMART ACTIONS TOMORROW

Lower your risk of urinary problems with these tips:

Go to the bathroom after sex. Urinate soon after having intercourse. This may help flush out bacteria that may have entered your urethra during sex. Cleansing your genital and anal areas before intercourse also may reduce your risk of getting a UTI.

Consider your birth control. Spermicides, diaphragms, cervical caps and unlubricated condoms all may irritate a woman's urethra or bladder. This may lead to a UTI. Avoid feminine hygiene sprays and douches. They also may cause irritation.

Dress right. Wear cotton underwear and loose-fitting clothes. This promotes air circulation. Tight undergarments and pants trap moisture and promote the growth of bacteria.

Stick with showers. Take showers instead of baths. This helps prevent bacteria from getting into your bladder. It also lowers the risk of irritation.

Take the next step. If you're prone to repeated UTIs, ask your doctor if taking preventive medicine may be a good choice for you.

Don't Live with Leakage

You don't have to live with bladder leakage—even if it's small or happens only when you laugh or cough. Don't wait until the leakage gets worse. Talk with your doctor. You may be able to treat it with lifestyle changes. Avoiding trigger foods may help. Women may benefit from doing daily Kegel exercises. Ask your doctor how.

VAGINAL DISCHARGE OR ITCH

UNDERSTANDING YOUR SYMPTOMS

The body has many ways of protecting itself. In women, vaginal discharge is one of those ways. A vaginal discharge is normal. It helps keep the vagina moist. Discharge also acts as a natural cleanser. It removes bacteria and germs, which may help prevent infections. Normal discharge is clear or slightly yellow, and thin in consistency. It occurs in small amounts.

On the other hand, abnormal vaginal discharge may look yellow, green, gray or white. It may be lumpy, like cottage cheese, or have a bad smell. It may cause itching or redness in the genital area. Abnormal vaginal discharge may be due to a bacterial or fungal infection. Other reasons for an abnormal discharge include a sexually transmitted disease (STD) or a pelvic infection. See Abdominal Pain, Page 84.

---

85 DECIDING YOUR NEXT STEP

SEEK EMERGENCY CARE:

- You're in severe pain.
- You have a new abnormal discharge, a fever of 100.4° F or higher, and pain or tenderness in the lower abdomen. You may also have nausea, vomiting, fatigue and body aches. Your pain may increase when you walk or move.
- You have a fever of 104° F or higher.
- You have intense shaking chills—more than just shivering.

(Continued)

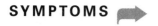

DECIDING YOUR NEXT STEP *(Continued)*

SEE YOUR DOCTOR TODAY:

- You've had an IUD inserted within the past month and are now having an unusual vaginal discharge.
- You have an area of skin near your vagina that's red, swollen, hot and tender, or painful.
- You have red streaks on your skin. Or, an area of your skin is draining a significant amount of pus.

CALL YOUR DOCTOR OR NURSE HELP LINE:

- You're pregnant and experience a change in the color, consistency or amount of your normal vaginal discharge.
- You have abnormal vaginal discharge.
- You have genital lesions, sores or blisters. Or, you have a new genital lump or wart.
- You suspect that you were exposed to a sexually transmitted disease.
- You've been taking a prescribed antibiotic for 48 hours. But, you've seen no improvement in your symptoms.
- Your genital itching, burning or discomfort persists. Or, it's a recurring problem.
- You have pain during intercourse.
- You tried self-care but it didn't work.

TRY SELF-CARE:

- You don't have abnormal discharge or odor. You don't have any of the symptoms described above.

SMART ACTIONS TODAY

If your symptoms indicate self-care:

Improve feminine hygiene. Change sanitary pads and tampons often. Choose unscented types. They're less likely to irritate. Don't use feminine hygiene sprays.

Try a sitz bath. Soak in only a few inches of warm water. Or, add half a cup of baking soda to a full, warm tub. Skip bubbles and soap. This may help ease discomfort. If you're pregnant, check with your doctor first.

SMART ACTIONS TOMORROW

Lifestyle choices may affect vaginal health. Keep in mind:

Protect yourself. If you're sexually active, you can help reduce your risk of STDs. Be sure to use a latex condom. If you're allergic to latex, use a polyurethane condom. Other birth control doesn't protect you from STDs.

Get tested. If you've been exposed to an STD, avoid sexual activity until after you have been diagnosed and treated—and your condition has cleared. Your partner also should be evaluated and treated, as necessary.

Have a checkup. Schedule a yearly gynecological exam. Ask about Pap smears and STD testing. See Health Screenings Women Need, Page 222.

MYTH OR TRUTH?

REGULAR DOUCHING IS HEALTHY

MYTH. Cleansing with douche disturbs the normal conditions in a healthy vagina. Douching may cause an existing infection to be pushed in deeper—into your uterus and even into your ovaries.

PART THREE

15
TAKE-CHARGE TOOLS

Get Equipped to Make Smart Choices

W E ALL UNDERSTAND WHAT TAKING CHARGE means in the workplace, on the sports field or when planning family matters. But, what does it mean in terms of health care? It means being informed and keeping good records. Preventing illnesses and being prepared for emergencies are part of it, too. And, don't forget about working effectively with your doctor. Sound difficult and time-consuming? It's easier than you think. The following pages are filled with tips, sample logs, personal medical records, screening charts and much more. Why not put these tools to work for you right away? And, be sure to share your notes with your doctor. Now, that's taking charge.

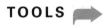

86 ▶ EMERGENCY CARE CONTACTS

Use this page to record important numbers. Post it next to your telephone. And, keep a copy in your purse or wallet. Be sure to update it as necessary.

Emergency: Call 911

Fire: _____

Police: _____

Other emergency medical services: _____

Poison control: 1-800-222-1222

Primary care doctor's name: _____

Office phone: _____

Emergency and after-hours number: _____

Other doctor's name: _____

Office phone: _____

Emergency and after-hours number: _____

Nurse help line: _____

Local personal emergency contact: _____

Phone: _____

Out-of-town personal emergency contact: _____

Phone: _____

Pharmacy name: _____

Phone: _____

Hospital name: _____

Phone: _____

Dentist's name: _____

Phone: _____

Health insurance company: _____

Policy number: _____

Group number: _____

Member service phone: _____

State public health department: _____

Animal control: _____

87 YOUR FIRST-AID KIT: THE ESSENTIALS

Keep the following basic supplies on hand to be prepared.

First-aid essentials:
- Adhesive bandages in a variety of sizes
- Antibiotic ointment to help prevent infections
- Antibiotic towelettes for disinfection
- A cleansing agent or soap
- Two pairs of latex or non-latex (if allergic) sterile gloves
- Sterile dressings to stop bleeding
- Eye wash solution
- Thermometer
- Triangular cloth bandages for slings
- Hydrocortisone cream and oral antihistamines

Additional supplies that may come in handy:
- Scissors and tweezers
- Aspirin and non-aspirin pain relievers
- Cold packs

If you have a baby in your household, keep extras of these items on hand:
- Formula
- Diapers
- Baby wipes
- Diaper rash ointment

Other supplies to stock up on—depending on your family's needs:
- Contact lenses and supplies; extra eyeglasses
- Denture needs
- Prescribed medications and medical supplies
- Personal hygiene items

Source: Adapted from *Ready America*, Department of Homeland Security

88 AT-A-GLANCE GUIDE TO OTC MEDICATIONS

Over-the-counter (OTC) medications are used to treat many ailments and symptoms. But, you must take them with care. Follow the package directions. Check with your doctor if you're pregnant or breast-feeding. When you're not sure if a certain medication is safe for you, be sure to ask your doctor. Here are some key safety tips:

Read the whole label. This will help you decide if the product is right for you. Pay attention to any warnings. Take note of any possible side effects or possible reactions.

Choose a product that treats only your symptoms. Also, don't combine medicines that have the same active ingredient. This may include OTC, prescription or multi-symptom medicines.

Follow directions. Take only the amount listed on the label. And, take it only as often as stated. Don't take OTC drugs longer than the label says, unless your doctor tells you to.

Learn what to avoid. Some OTC drugs may cause side effects or reactions. Drowsiness and rashes are two examples. Or, they may not work when taken with other OTC or prescription medications. Dietary supplements and certain foods or alcohol may also work against OTC drugs. And, some OTC drugs may change how other medications are absorbed. Ask your doctor or pharmacist if you're not sure.

Pregnant? Women who are pregnant or trying to become pregnant should speak with their doctors before taking any OTC medications. This applies to women who are breast-feeding, too.

Don't assume. Be sure to read the label and instructions every time you open a new package. Something may have changed since the last time you bought that product. Maybe the strength is different. Or, perhaps an ingredient changed.

Check expiration dates. Drugs start to lose effectiveness after their expiration dates. They may even become toxic. Read the label for the right way to dispose of the medicine. If there are no instructions, you can try this: Remove the medicine from its original container. Then, mix it with used coffee grounds or kitty litter. Or, mix it with foul-smelling garbage. Place the mixture in a sealed container. Then, put it in the trash.

COMMON OTC MEDICATIONS

PAIN RELIEVERS

There are two main types of OTC pain relievers: nonsteroidal anti-inflammatory drugs (NSAIDs) and acetaminophen. NSAIDs include aspirin, ibuprofen and naproxen. They block the body from making natural chemicals that cause pain. They help lower fever and inflammation. And, aspirin may help prevent blood clots. Acetaminophen changes how the body perceives pain. It also helps lower fever.

Aspirin

Used for: Lowering fever and easing mild to moderate pain caused by muscle aches and stiffness. Aspirin and other NSAIDs also may help bring down inflammation. Doctors may also recommend aspirin for those at risk of cardiovascular disease. Taking aspirin raises the chance of bleeding. Long-term use may cause gastrointestinal problems or ulcers in some people. Taking enteric-coated aspirin may lessen stomach irritation for some people. Taking it with food and milk helps, too. *Caution:* Never give aspirin to anyone younger than age 19. It's linked to a rare but sometimes fatal condition called Reye's syndrome.

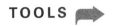
Ibuprofen and Naproxen

Used for: Relieving pain and lowering fever. Like aspirin, these NSAIDs may ease the redness and swelling of inflammation. For some people, they're easier on the stomach than aspirin. However, they may cause stomach discomfort and/or ulceration. So, take them with food or milk. *Caution:* Taking ibuprofen for pain relief may lower the benefits of taking aspirin for the heart, if you take these two OTC medications at the same time. Talk with your doctor about the best time of day to take each of these for the best result.

NSAIDs Caution: Talk with your doctor before taking any NSAIDs—including aspirin—if you're taking any prescriptions. If you're older than age 60, have a history of stomach ulcers or bleeding problems, or have another medical condition, you should check with your doctor first.

Acetaminophen

Used for: Bringing down fever and easing mild to moderate pain from a number of ailments and conditions. It's thought to be a safe alternative to aspirin for people who have various health concerns. It seldom causes stomach problems. And, it doesn't cause bleeding. Talk with your doctor before taking it if you have kidney or liver disease. Also, consult your doctor first if you have three or more alcoholic drinks every day.

HEARTBURN MEDICATIONS

Antacids, proton pump inhibitors and acid blockers

Used for: Relief of heartburn, also known as acid reflux disease or gastroesophageal reflux. Talk with your doctor if you have heartburn often. If you have a chronic condition, such as kidney disease, or take other medicines, check with your doctor first.

COLDS AND ALLERGY MEDICATIONS

Talk with your doctor or pharmacist before taking any OTC cold or allergy medications if you have a chronic health condition or take other medications.

Antihistamines

Used for: Prevention and treatment of allergy symptoms. This includes sneezing, itchy and watery eyes, or a runny nose. They also help stop the itchiness caused by insect bites, poison ivy and poison oak, or other allergic reactions. These drugs may cause drowsiness. When taken for lengthy periods of time, they may not work as well.

Decongestants

Used for: Relieving a stuffed-up nose caused by a cold, the flu, sinusitis or allergies. Limit the use of decongestant nose sprays and drops to no more than three days in a row. Your body may become dependent on them.

Antihistamines and Decongestants Caution: These medications, used separately or in combination, may be harmful for older men who have an enlarged prostate.

A Note about Medications for Children

Children need medications and dosage amounts based on age and weight. Be certain that you give the correct dose. Never let children take medicine without supervision.

Some studies have shown that OTC cough and cold medicines don't treat symptoms in children younger than age 6. In fact, they may pose serious risks. Currently, the FDA says do not use these medicines at all for children younger than age 2. What about children age 2 and older? For safety's sake, you must ask your doctor what's right for your child. This issue continues to be studied at the time of printing and these recommendations may change.

---

89 ➤ YOUR MEDICATION RECORD

Make copies of this form. Keep one in your wallet or purse. Tape one inside a kitchen or bathroom cabinet. Don't forget to keep a copy in your car. Always bring it with you when you visit your doctor. List all the medications you take. Include prescriptions, over-the-counter medicines, vitamins and herbs. It's also wise to make note of all medication allergies.

Medication or supplement: _____

Reason for taking: _____

Dose and frequency: _____

Prescribed by: _____

Date started: _____

Medication or supplement: _____

Reason for taking: _____

Dose and frequency: _____

Prescribed by: _____

Date started: _____

Medication or supplement: _____

Reason for taking: _____

Dose and frequency: _____

Prescribed by: _____

Date started: _____

Medication or supplement: _____

Reason for taking: _____

Dose and frequency: _____

Prescribed by: _____

Date started: _____

90 ▸ SYMPTOM CHECKLIST

The more prepared you are for each doctor visit, the better. The tools below may help. Make a copy of this checklist. Use it before your next appointment. Be sure to add your own concerns, too.

Things to jot down before your next doctor visit:
- What are your symptoms?
- When did they start and how often do they occur?
- Does anything make them better or worse?
- What prescriptions are you taking? List OTC medications and supplements (including herbal), too.
- Have there been any recent changes in your life that may be contributing to your symptoms?

Notes: _____

_____

_____

Questions for your health care professional:
- What causes these symptoms/this condition?
- Could any drugs I'm taking be contributing to the problem?
- Should I take any OTC medications to help treat my symptoms?
- How is this condition treated? Are any tests needed?
- Will there be any side effects from the treatment?
- How long until I see results from the treatment?
- Is this a condition that may require surgery?
- Do I need to limit my diet or my activities?
- What can I do on my own to ease my symptoms?
- How can I prevent this condition in the future?
- Are there any support groups for this condition?
- Where can I get more information?
- Should I come back for a follow-up visit? If so, when?

Notes: _____

_____

_____

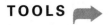

91 YOUR MEDICAL HISTORY

It's important for your doctor to know your medical history. It may be used to help make a diagnosis or determine the best treatment for you. Use this form to create a personal health record. Your employer or health plan may offer similar tools. Update this form every year or if your health conditions change.

Blood Type _____

Allergies

Medication/Substance	Reaction
_____	_____
_____	_____
_____	_____
_____	_____

Chronic Conditions

Condition	Date Diagnosed	Treatment
_____	_____	_____
_____	_____	_____
_____	_____	_____
_____	_____	_____

Surgeries

Surgery	Date
_____	_____
_____	_____
_____	_____

Prosthetics, Implants, Pacemakers, Defibrillators, etc.

Device	Date
_____	_____
_____	_____
_____	_____
_____	_____

For Women, Gynecologic and Obstetric History
(Include things such as pregnancies, problems with periods, onset of menopause, etc.)

What   Date

_____   _____
_____   _____
_____   _____

Past Medical History

Illness   Date

_____   _____
_____   _____
_____   _____

Most Recent Immunizations

For more information, visit the Centers for Disease Control and Prevention at www.cdc.gov/vaccines/.

Immunization   Date

Hepatitis A   _____
Hepatitis B   _____
Influenza (flu shot or nasal vaccine)   _____
MMR* (measles-mumps-rubella)   _____
Pneumonia   _____
Meningitis   _____
Tetanus   _____
Varicella* (chicken pox) shot   _____
Tdap (tetanus, diphtheria and pertussis)
*If you have a reliable history of having had this disease, record the date here.

Most Recent Screenings

For recommended screenings by gender, see Pages 220 and 222.

Screening   Date   Result

_____   _____   _____
_____   _____   _____
_____   _____   _____
_____   _____   _____

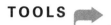

92 ▶ YOUR FAMILY HEALTH HISTORY

You may think that your uncle had lung cancer just because he was a smoker. Or, that your mother's depression was a one-time event. The fact is, these and other pieces of your family's medical history could help save your life. Families share genes. But, they also share some lifestyle behaviors, such as eating habits. Even the tendency to smoke is often passed down. Family members may also share similar environmental exposures. The more you know about your family's health history, the better.

Family Member's Name			
Relationship to You[1]			
Still Living?[2]			
Heart Disease			
Hypertension			
Stroke			
Diabetes			
Colon Cancer			
Breast Cancer			
Ovarian Cancer			
Other Diseases/Notes			

[1] Include only blood relatives.
[2] If deceased, include age and cause of death.
Source: Adapted from the United States Department of Health & Human Services

Why not create your own family medical history? Make copies of the chart below to gather the information. Or, use the interactive tool found at www.familyhistory.hhs.gov. Keep in mind, this chart is not a complete list of inherited diseases. You may need to add conditions that apply to your family. Be sure to share the information with your doctor. And, make copies for your entire family. You'll all benefit. Set aside time each year to update the history.

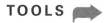

93 ▶ HEALTH SCREENINGS MEN NEED

Preventive screenings may help you stay healthy. Talk
with your doctor about which screenings you may need
and how often you should have them. Also, check
coverage with your health plan.

SCREENING	CHECKS FOR
Abdominal aortic aneurysm	Enlarged aorta (major blood vessel from heart) in your abdomen
Blood glucose testing	Type 2 diabetes
Blood pressure	High blood pressure
Cholesterol	High cholesterol
Colonoscopy and other colon tests	Colorectal cancer
Digital rectal exam	Abnormalities of the prostate
HIV test	Human immunodeficiency virus
Prostate-specific antigen (PSA) test	High levels of PSA in the blood, which may indicate a problem with the prostate
STD screening	Sexually transmitted diseases, such as gonorrhea, syphilis and chlamydia

Onetime screening if you're between ages 65 and 75 and have ever smoked.

• If your blood pressure is above 135/80.
• If you're 45 or older, or if you're younger than 45 and overweight.
• Repeat every three years, if results are normal.

At least every two years, starting at age 18.

Uniform screening recommendations have not been set. However, consider checking your cholesterol regularly starting at age 35, or at age 20 if:
• You have a family history of early heart disease.
• You have high blood pressure or diabetes.
• You smoke.

Start at age 50—or younger if you have a family history of the disease or other risk factors. Talk with your doctor about the test and frequency that's right for you.

Uniform screening recommendations have not been set. Talk with your doctor about whether you need a screening.

The Centers for Disease Control and Prevention recommends voluntary testing of any patients in health care facilities (doctors' offices, hospitals) and annual testing for at-risk people. You are at increased risk if:
• You are being treated for a sexually transmitted disease.
• You had a blood transfusion between 1978 and 1985.
• You have past or present sexual partners who are HIV positive, bisexual or use intravenous drugs.
• You have had sex with men since 1975.
• You have had unprotected sex with multiple partners.
• You have used or are now using intravenous drugs.

Uniform screening recommendations have not been set. Talk with your doctor about whether you need a screening.

Talk with your doctor about whether you need a screening.

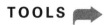

94 HEALTH SCREENINGS WOMEN NEED

Preventive screenings may help you stay healthy. Talk with your doctor about which screenings you may need and how often you should have them. Also, check coverage with your health plan.

SCREENING	CHECKS FOR
Blood glucose testing	Type 2 diabetes
Blood pressure	High blood pressure
Bone-density test	Osteoporosis
Chlamydia screening	Chlamydia
Cholesterol	High cholesterol
Clinical breast exams	Breast cancer
Colonoscopy and other colon tests	Colorectal cancer
HIV test	Human immunodeficiency virus

WHEN TO HAVE

- If your blood pressure is above 135/80.
- If you're 45 or older, or if you're younger than 45 and overweight.
- Repeat every three years, if results are normal.

At least every two years, starting at age 18.

Regularly beginning at age 65, or between the ages of 60 and 64 if you weigh 154 pounds or less or if you have other individual risk factors—such as smoking, weight loss, family history of osteoporosis, decreased physical activity, alcohol or caffeine use, or low calcium and vitamin D intake.

If you're 25 or younger and sexually active. Also, if you are at an increased risk, you should be screened no matter what your age. Increased risk factors include having new or multiple sexual partners, a partner who is not monogamous, inconsistent condom use or having had an STD in the past.

Uniform screening recommendations have not been set. However, consider checking your cholesterol regularly starting at age 45, or at age 20 if:
- You have a family history of early heart disease.
- You have high blood pressure or diabetes.
- You smoke.

Experts disagree on the value of clinical breast exams. Speak to your doctor regarding the breast cancer screening program that's right for you.

Start at age 50—or younger if you have a family history of the disease, or other risk factors. Talk with your doctor about the test and frequency that's right for you.

The Centers for Disease Control and Prevention recommends voluntary testing of any patients in health care facilities (doctors' offices, hospitals) and annual testing for at-risk people. You are at increased risk if:
- You are being treated for a sexually transmitted disease.
- You had a blood transfusion between 1978 and 1985.
- You have past or present sexual partners who are HIV positive, bisexual or use intravenous drugs.
- You have had unprotected sex with multiple partners.
- You have used or are now using intravenous drugs.
Note: The United States Preventive Services Task Force also recommends screening of all pregnant women for HIV.

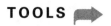

HEALTH SCREENINGS WOMEN NEED
(Continued)

SCREENING	CHECKS FOR
Mammogram	Breast cancer
Pap test	Cervical cancer
STD screening	Sexually transmitted diseases, such as gonorrhea and syphilis

- Every one to two years starting at age 40.
- The American Cancer Society recommends a yearly mammogram and MRI starting at age 30 for high-risk patients.

Initial screening at age 21 or within three years of becoming sexually active, whichever comes first. Most experts recommend pap smears and pelvic exams every one to three years thereafter. Speak to your doctor regarding the screening schedule that's right for you.

Talk with your doctor about whether you need a screening.

95 ➤ YOUR HEALTHFUL WEIGHT

Body mass index (BMI) and waist-to-hip ratio are tools for determining your body fat. They'll give you a good idea of whether you are underweight, normal weight, overweight or obese. Wondering if your weight is putting you at a greater risk of health problems? Don't guess. Have a talk with your doctor.

To find your BMI:

Your BMI is based on your height and weight. Use the chart below to see where you stand. Or, use the BMI calculator from the National Heart, Lung and Blood Institute at www.nhlbisupport.com/bmi.

BMI	21	22	23	24	25	26	27	28	29	30	31
HEIGHT (inches)	BODY WEIGHT (pounds)										
60	107	112	118	123	128	133	138	143	148	153	158
61	111	116	122	127	132	137	143	148	153	158	164
62	115	120	126	131	136	142	147	153	158	164	169
63	118	124	130	135	141	146	152	158	163	169	175
64	122	128	134	140	145	151	157	163	169	174	180
65	126	132	138	144	150	156	162	168	174	180	186
66	130	136	142	148	155	161	167	173	179	186	192
67	134	140	146	153	159	166	172	178	185	191	198
68	138	144	151	158	164	171	177	184	190	197	203
69	142	149	155	162	169	176	182	189	196	203	209
70	146	153	160	167	174	181	188	195	202	209	216
71	150	157	165	172	179	186	193	200	208	215	222
72	154	162	169	177	184	191	199	206	213	221	228
73	159	166	174	182	189	197	204	212	219	227	235

The shaded area indicates the overweight range. Anything 30 and above is considered obese.

What the BMI numbers mean:
Underweight = Less than 18.5
Normal weight = 18.5 to 24.9
Overweight = 25 to 29.9
Obese = 30 or more

- It's possible to have a high BMI and low body fat. This is true for many highly trained athletes.

- BMI for children and teenagers is viewed differently. It takes gender and age into account. BMI is also interpreted differently for those ages 65 and older.

To figure out your waist-to-hip ratio:
People who carry more weight around the waist have a higher risk of health problems. Research has shown this to be the case. To find your waist-to-hip ratio, grab a tape measure. Start with your hips. Measure around the widest part of your buttocks. Then, wrap the tape around the smallest part of your waist. This is usually just above the belly button. Divide your waist measurement by your hip measurement.

You're at a higher risk of heart disease and other health conditions if you have these results:
- Women—ratio is greater than 0.85
- Men—ratio is greater than 0.9

96 ➤ M<small>Y</small>PYRAMID FOR FOOD CHOICES

MyPyramid.gov has personalized eating plans to help you make smart food choices. Visit the site for more details.

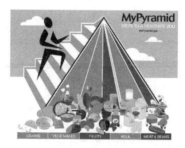

Grains: Eat 3 ounces or more of whole-grain foods each day. Bread, cereal and pasta are some examples. Check ingredient lists to see that the word *whole* is before the grain name.

Vegetables: Eat more dark-green vegetables, orange vegetables, and dry beans and peas.

Fruit: Whether fresh, frozen, canned or dried, get a good variety. Think beyond apples, oranges and bananas.

Milk: Eat low-fat or fat-free dairy products. Lactose-free products or other calcium sources fit here, too.

Meats and beans: Choose low-fat or lean meats and poultry. Fish, peas, beans, nuts and seeds are also key. When cooking, it's best to bake, broil or grill your meats.

Oils: There is such a thing as healthful fats. They're found in fish, nuts and vegetable oils. Make the most of these choices. Try to avoid solid fats whenever possible. This includes butter, stick margarine and shortening,

Discretionary calories: These are the additional calories you may "spend" once you've satisfied your body's essential nutrient needs. These might be extras such as salad dressings or syrup.

YOUR DIET JOURNAL

A food diary may give you insights into what and how much you eat. It may help you and your doctor tailor your diet to your health needs. Make a copy of this form. Use it for a week or two. Or, ask your doctor how long you should track your eating habits.

What I Ate Today

Jot down everything you eat and drink. Be specific. And, be honest. Include any extras, such as salad dressings and beverages. Also, try to estimate the size of each portion.

Breakfast: _____

_____

_____

Lunch: _____

_____

_____

Dinner: _____

_____

_____

Snacks: _____

_____

_____

Notes

Write down notes such as your mood while eating. Also, include where you ate and with whom.

_____

_____

_____

Source: Adapted from the American Academy of Family Physicians

98 ▶ YOUR ACTIVITY LOG

It can be hard to know just how much movement you're getting during each week. Tracking your activity is a great idea. Jot down how you felt while being active. Then, note how you felt at the end of each day. Over time, you'll be able to see how far you've come in meeting your fitness goals.

My Activities Today

Write down your daily activities here. Remember, all movement counts. You probably do more than you realize—gardening, housework, that walk to the coffee shop. Did you take the stairs instead of the elevator? Jot that down, too.

Morning: _____

_____

_____

_____

Afternoon: _____

_____

_____

_____

Evening: _____

_____

_____

_____

Total activity (minutes): _____

Notes: _____

_____

_____

_____

99 CALORIES BURNED
DURING ACTIVITIES

Here's a look at how some simple activities add up in terms of calories burned. Compare them to sitting and watching TV, which burns just 68 calories per hour.

Activity	Calories burned per hour*
Aerobics	480
Biking (more than 10 mph)	590
Dancing	330
Gardening/light yard work	330
Heavy yard work	440
Hiking	370
Jogging (5 mph)	590
Playing with kids	216
Stretching	180
Swimming (slow laps)	510
Walking (briskly, 3.5 mph)	280
Weight lifting (light workout)	220

* For a 154-pound person. Source: U.S. Dept. of Health & Human Services

100 10 SNACKS UNDER 100 CALORIES

Here's a list of smart snack foods to keep near your fridge.

Food	Calories
½ cup raw baby carrots	30
1 cup plain popcorn	31
17 grapes	57
18 pistachio nuts	70
1 part-skim string-cheese stick	72
2 tablespoons hummus on ¼ whole-wheat pita bread	89
1 small banana	90
½ cup fat-free vanilla ice cream	93
11 baked tortilla chips with 3 tablespoons salsa	95
½ English muffin with 1 teaspoon peanut butter	97

INDEX

A

abdominal aortic aneurysm screenings, 220
abdominal pain, 84–87
abdominal strength, 195
accident prevention. See safety precautions
acetaminophen, 212. See also pain relievers
acid reflux disease, 212
activity log, 230
aerobic workouts, 29
affection, 43
air travel, 134
alcohol consumption. See also rubbing alcohol
  depression and, 127
  fainting and, 139
  heart health and, 113
  heart rate and, 184
  medications and, 61–62, 127
  travel safety and, 81
  wellness and, 61–62
allergies
  breathing problems from, 100-102
  medicines for, 213
  nasal congestion from, 167
  nosebleeds from, 174
  rashes from, 185
Alzheimer's disease, 23
anaphylaxis, 100, 152-153
anemia, 136
anger management, 39–40, 46
angina, 110, 112–113
animal bites, 88–90
ankles, sprained, 192
antacids, 212
anthocyanin, 23
antibiotics, 170, 190
antidepressant medications, 127

antihistamines
  for allergies, 101
  described, 213
  for insect bites and stings, 154
  for nasal congestion, 169
  for rashes, 187
  use caution, 213
anxiety, 91–93
aortic dissection, 110
appendicitis, 84
arthritis, 156–159
aspirin. See also pain relievers
  described, 211
  for toothaches, 123
  use caution, 96, 211
asthma
  described, 100
  effects of, 100, 114
  treatment of, 102, 116
autoimmune diseases, 163

B

back injuries, 178, 195
back pain, low, 94–97
bad breath
  causes of, 121
  with other symptoms, 122
baking soda bath, 197
barley, 21
barotrauma, 132
baths. See showers and baths
batteries, safe use of, 109
beans and legumes
  in MyPyramid, 228
  as protein source, 15
  in vegetarian diet, 17
beds and bedding
  back pain and, 97
  dust mites and, 170
bipolar disorder, 125

birth control,
  UTIs and, 202
black widow spiders, 152
bladder leakage, 202
blisters, from burns, 108, 197
blood clots, 111
blood pressure
  connectedness and, 50
  dizziness and, 129
  exercise and, 27, 35, 48
  food choices and, 24
  heart health and, 113
  screenings, 220, 222
  sodium and, 18
  stress and, 36
  weight control and, 25
blood pressure medications, 28, 117
blood sugar levels
  in diabetics, 113, 139
  headaches and, 147
blood sugar screenings, 220, 222
body mass index (BMI), 226–227. See also weight control
bone-density tests, 222
bone health. See bone injuries, extremities; osteoporosis prevention
bone injuries, extremities, 98-99
breast exams, 222
breathing exercises, 40, 102
breathing problems, 100-103
bronchitis, 114
brown recluse spiders, 152
brown rice, 21
bruises, 104–105
burns, 106–109. See also sunburn
butter, for burns, 109
B vitamins, 19

INDEX ➡

C

caffeine
  headaches and, 147
  heart rate and, 184
  sleep and, 59
  travel and, 81
calamine lotion, 154, 187
calcium. See also milk
  daily intake of, 19
  joint pain and, 159
  sources of, 24
calories
  counting, 24
  discretionary, 228
  number burned by
    activity, 231
  snacks under 100
    calories, 231
cancer
  exercise and, 29
  food choices and, 21, 23
  smoking and, 62
carbohydrates, 12–13
carbon monoxide
  poisoning, 69–70
car maintenance, 78–79
carpal tunnel syndrome
  assembly line, and, 180,
    181
  computers and, 180
  described, 178
  splints for, 181
car trouble, safety and, 76
cat bites, 88, 89
cell phones, 76, 78
checklists. See forms and
  checklists
chemical burns, 106–109
chest pain, 110–113
chewing tobacco, 124
chicken soup, as remedy,
  149
children
  aspirin use caution, 96
  honey use caution, 117
  medications for, 213
chlamydia screenings, 222
cholesterol, in foods, 14

cholesterol levels
  connectedness and, 50
  exercise and, 27
  food choices and, 14, 15,
    17, 21, 24
  heart health and, 113
  screenings, 220, 222
  weight control and, 25
chronic obstructive
  pulmonary disease
  (COPD)
  effects of, 100, 114
  smoking and, 103
  treatments for, 102
cluster headaches, 144
cold medicines, 169, 213
colds
  nosebleeds from, 174
  preventing, 103, 177
  symptoms of, 167
cold treatments
  back pain, 96
  bruises, 105
  contraindications, 109
  groin strain, 161
  headaches, 146
  muscle pain, 165
  numbness and tingling,
    180
  sprains, 194
  sunburn, 197
colonoscopy, 220, 222
community involvement,
  47–49
computer use, 180, 181
connectedness
  anxiety and, 93
  community, 47–49
  friends, 45–47
  longevity and, 42
  marriage, 43–44
  pets, 50
constipation, 13
COPD. See chronic
  obstructive pulmonary
  disease
core strength, 195
corn, 21

cosmetics, sun sensitivity
  and, 198
costochondritis, 110
coughs, 114–117, 213
cough suppressants, 116
cranberry juice, for UTIs,
  201
cuts, 118–120

D

daily activities, as exercise,
  31, 32, 33, 34
daily values (DVs), 18
dairy products. See milk
dancing, as exercise, 29
decongestants, 169, 177,
  213
dehydration. See also fluid
  intake; water
  dizziness from, 129
  fainting from, 136, 137
  fevers and, 140, 141
  from vomiting, 171–173
dental problems, 121–124
depression
  connectedness and, 45
  management of, 41–42,
    125–128
  sleep deprivation and, 58
  types of, 125
diabetes
  alcohol use and, 61
  blood sugar and, 113,
    139
  cold treatment caution,
    96
  exercise and, 27, 29
  food choices and, 13, 21
  sleep and, 58
  symptoms of, 199
  weight control and, 25
diaries, as diagnostic tool
  abdominal pain, 87
  headaches, 147
  nausea and vomiting,
    173
diarrhea, 81

INDEX ➡

INDEX ➡

exercise, 27
food choices, 24
ovarian cysts, 84
over-the-counter drugs,
210–213. See also
medications; medication
side effects; specific
types

P

pain relievers, as treatment
alcohol use and, 62
back pain, 96
bruises, 105
fevers, 142
influenza, 149
joint pain, 158
male genital pain, 162
muscle pain, 112, 165
nasal congestion, 169
numbness and tingling,
180
sore throats, 191
sprains, 194
sunburn, 197
toothaches, 123
types of, 211–212
pancreatitis, 84
panic disorder, 91
pap tests, 224
penile pain or problems,
160–162
peptic ulcers, 85
pericarditis, 110
periodontal disease, 121
periodontitis, 124
personal health record,
216–217
personal safety, 75–76
pets, 50, 90
pharmacists, 55
physical therapy, 194
physician assistants, 55
pleurisy, 111
PMDD, 125
pneumonia, 111

pneumothorax, 111
poison ivy, 185
polyunsaturated fats, 14
portion control, 25
postpartum depression
(PPD), 125
post-traumatic stress
disorder (PTSD), 91
potassium, 19
poultry, 16
PPD, 125
praise, of spouse, 44
pregnancy, medications
and, 210
premenstrual dysphoric
disorder (PMDD), 125
prescription drugs. See
medications; medication
side effects; specific
types
prostate-specific antigen
(PSA) test, 220
protein, 15–17
PSA test, 220
PTSD, 91
pulmonary embolism, 111
puncture wounds, 120

Q

quinoa, 21

R

RA, 156
rapid heartbeat, 182–184
rashes, 185–188
Recommended Daily
Intakes (RDIs), 19
rectal exams, 220
relaxation techniques
anger management, 40
anxiety management, 93
stress management, 38
religion, 49
repetitive motion disorders,
163. See also carpal
tunnel syndrome

repetitive movement,
numbness from, 181
rest, as treatment
coughs, 116
influenza, 149
joint pain, 158
muscle pain, 165
numbness and tingling,
181
sore throats, 191
restless leg syndrome, 60
resveratrol, 23
Reye's syndrome, 96
rheumatoid arthritis (RA),
156
rice, brown, 21
RICE formula, 194
rubbing alcohol, for fevers,
142

S

SAD (seasonal affective
disorder), 125
SAD (social anxiety
disorder), 91
safety precautions
burn prevention, 109
carbon monoxide
poisoning, 69–70
driving habits, 77–79
fall prevention, 195
fire prevention, 66–69
first-aid kits, 76, 209
food poisoning, 70–74
germs, 74
personal safety, 75–76
travel, 80–81
saline gargle, 191
saturated fats, 14
scuba diving, 135
seasonal affective disorder
(SAD), 125
seat belt use, 77
secondary headaches, 144
seeds and nuts, 17
septic arthritis, 156
sexual activity

INDEX

vegetarian diets, 17
vertigo, 129
visualization, 40
vitamin A, 19
vitamin C, 19
vitamin D, 19, 159
vitamins and minerals,
   18–19
vitamin supplements, 23
volunteering, 49

W

waist-to-hip ratio, 227. See
   also weight control
walking, 29, 75
water, 20, 30. See also
   dehydration; fluid intake
Web sites. See Internet
   tools
weight control
   benefits of, 25
   calorie requirements for,
   24
   exercise and, 27, 32
   healthful weight
   calculation, 226–227
   joint pain and, 159
   portion control for, 25
   tips for, 25–26
West Nile virus, 152, 153
whole grains, 20–21, 228
whole wheat, 21

Y

yoga, 48, 128
yogurt, 87